The Road to Good Nutrition

The Road to Good Nutrition

Editors

Manfred Eggersdorfer

Klaus Kraemer

Marie Ruel

Marc Van Ameringen

Hans Konrad Biesalski

Martin Bloem

Junshi Chen

Asma Lateef

Venkatesh Mannar

Kaiseraugust

183 figures and 14 tables, 2013

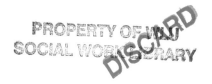
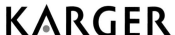
KARGER

Basel · Freiburg · Paris · London · New York · New Delhi · Bangkok
Beijing · Tokyo · Kuala Lumpur · Singapore · Sydney

Manfred Eggersdorfer
DSM Nutritional Products Ltd
Wurmisweg 576, 4303 Kaiseraugst, Switzerland

Klaus Kraemer
Sight and Life
P.O. Box 2116, Basel, CH-4002, Switzerland

Marie Ruel
IFPRI (International Food Policy Research Institute)
2033 K St, NW, Washington, DC 20006-1002, USA

Marc Van Ameringen
GAIN (Global Alliance for Improved Nutrition)
P.O. Box 55, 1211 Geneva 20, Switzerland

Hans Konrad Biesalski
Universität Hohenheim
Garbenstrasse 30, Bio I, 70593 Stuttgart, Germany

Martin Bloem
WFP (World Food Programme)
Via C.G. Viola 68,Parco dei Medici, 00148 Roma, Italy

Junshi Chen
National Institute of Nutrition & Food Safety,
Chinese Center for Disease Control & Prevention
155 Changbai Road, Changping District, 102206, P.R. China

Asma Lateef
Bread for the World Institute
425 3rd Street SW, Suite 1200, Washington, DC 20024, USA

Venkatesh Mannar
Micronutrient Initiative
180 Elgin Street, Suite 1000, Ottawa, Ontario, K2P 2K3, Canada

Library of Congress Cataloging-in-Publication Data

The road to good nutrition / editor, Manfred Eggersdorfer ... [et al.]
p. ; cm.
Includes bibliographical references and index.
ISBN 978-3-318-02549-1 (hard cover : alk. paper)
ISBN 978-3-318-02550-7 (e-ISBN)
I. Eggersdorfer, Manfred.
[DNLM: 1. Nutrition Policy. 2. Malnutrition. 3. World Health. QU 145.72]
RA645.N87
362.1963'9--dc23   2013031089

Copyright 2013 by S. Karger AG, P.O. Box, CH–4009 Basel (Switzerland)

www.karger.com

Printed in Germany on acid-free and non-aging paper (ISO 9706) by Kraft Druck, Ettlingen
ISBN 978-3-318-02549-1
e-ISBN 978-3-318-02550-7

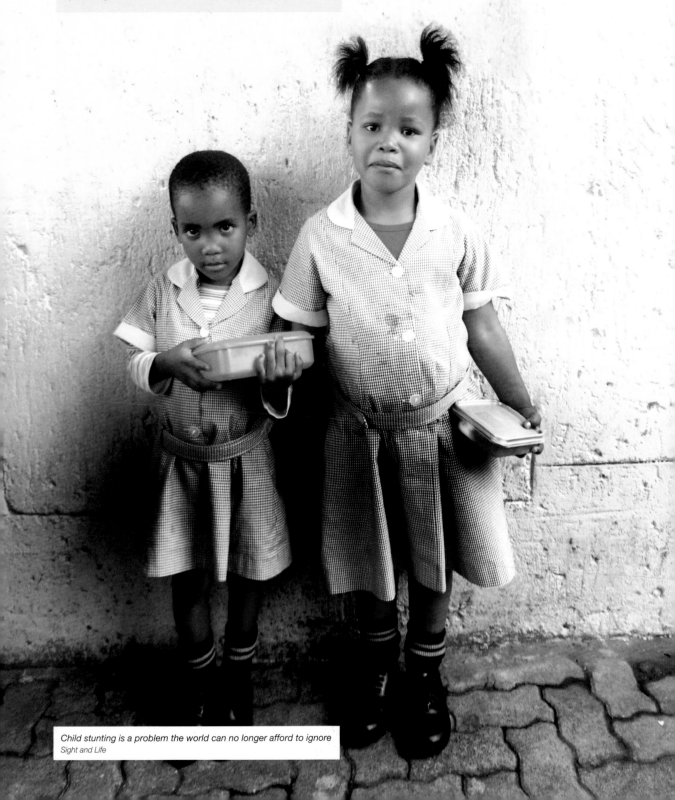

"Globally, 165 million children under age 5 are stunted as a result of malnutrition. This is the face of poverty,"

Jim Yong Kim, *President of the World Bank Group*

Child stunting is a problem the world can no longer afford to ignore
Sight and Life

Foreword

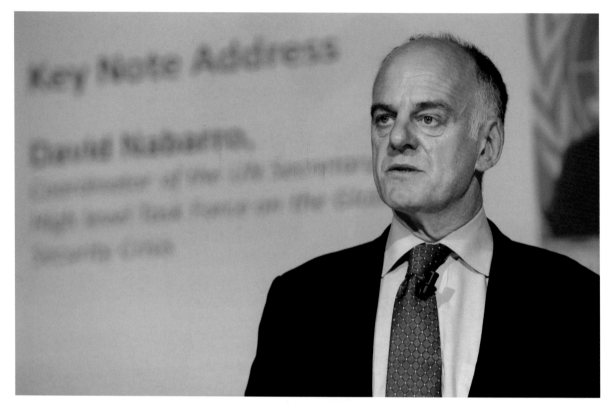

Dr David Nabarro

Special Representative of the UN Secretary-
General for Food Security and Nutrition
SUN Movement Coordinator

Working Together for Improved Nutrition

Approximately a third of the world's children face lifelong
economic and social disadvantage because of poor nutrition
during pregnancy and in the first two years of life. A
significant proportion of these children are disadvantaged
because of unbalanced diets that lead to obesity and its
associated health challenges. Malnutrition is a phenomenon
with many aspects, not all of them immediately apparent.

Analysis of efforts to tackle malnutrition conducted by The
Lancet originally in 2008 and again in 2013 indicates that a
range of specific interventions exist that can help people
enjoy good nutritional status. Experience shows that they
are most effective if national development strategies are
sensitive to the underlying determinants of people's
nutritional status.

> *"A person who has food has many
> problems. A person who has no
> food has only one problem."*
>
> **Chinese saying**

Nutrition-sensitive solutions

Since 2008 many governments, civil society organizations, research groups and intergovernmental agencies (including those within the United Nations system) have sought ways to scale up effective actions for better nutrition. The collective experience to date suggests that such efforts are successful if all the different groups that seek to enable improvements in people's nutrition work *together* in support of sound national policies, the implementation of effective interventions, and sector programs that are sensitive to the determinants of malnutrition.

The evidence also indicates that as efforts are made to scale up success, all the groups that seek to support the implementation of national policies should work in synergy. As they do so, they should, at all times, take account of the day-to-day challenges faced by communities at risk of malnutrition, aligning their efforts to promote social justice and nutritional equity, and monitoring their collective impact. Their overarching aim should be to enable all women and children – and their families – to realize their right to food and good nutrition.

A bold new way of collective and harmonized thinking

The *Scaling Up Nutrition* or *'SUN' Movement* was launched in September 2010 in response to the release earlier that year, by more than 100 national and international organizations, of the *Framework for Scaling Up Nutrition*.

The Movement is designed to bring together diverse stakeholders – central and local governments, civil society organizations, research groups and intergovernmental agencies and business enterprises – so that they can jointly work on improvements in nutrition on a scale that reflects the urgency and seriousness of the issue.

The SUN Movement embodies a bold new way of collective and harmonized thinking, action and communication for improved nutrition. It is specifically a movement, and not a new program, institution or fund. Through the Movement, national governments – both individually and jointly – are leading the worldwide effort to yield lasting nutritional benefits for individuals and societies within their respective countries. When joining the SUN Movement, they each commit to enabling people to access proven and innovative solutions for better nutrition, and to work in ways that increase the effectiveness of their investments so as to yield sustainable and equitable results.

The imperative to act

The Road to Good Nutrition is an expression of this new way of thinking. It brings together the experience and insights of globally recognized experts in the field of nutrition to create an in-depth introduction to the subject for the non-expert. This book is detailed, accurate and as up to date as possible, given the speed at which nutrition research on the one hand and nutrition policy on the other are evolving. The world of nutrition is moving fast, and it needs to, for the challenges we face are huge, and the imperative to act, overwhelming.

My hope is that *The Road to Good Nutrition* will help us all to accelerate our progress along the path to a world where everyone receives the food and the nutrition to which they have a self-evident right.

David Nabarro

Special Representative of the UN Secretary-General for Food Security and Nutrition

SUN Movement Coordinator

Rome, June 2013

Preface

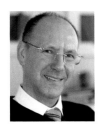

Manfred Eggersdorfer
SVP DSM Nutrition Science & Advocacy

The Road to Good Nutrition is about a journey. It is not the journey of a lone individual, or organization, or country, or even continent. It is a journey that the world has embarked on – and which we can only complete if we all walk the road together. This book is about how to improve the nutritional status of the world's population as a whole. It therefore touches each and every one of us, and we each have a role to play in helping the world a step further towards that goal.

This work is published at a critical moment in our global understanding of the challenges and opportunities we face. The need for a concerted approach to the elimination of malnutrition worldwide has never been greater. Nor has the world's desire to confront malnutrition in a concerted manner. The Scaling Up Nutrition (SUN) Movement continues to gather momentum even as this book goes to press; the evidential base for action has been strengthened yet further by the publication of the 2013 Lancet series on Maternal and Child Nutrition; and the interactions between nutritionists, policy-makers, program managers and donors have never been so many, so frequent or so productive. This is a moment which the world must seize. And to seize that moment, we must grasp the fact that, for all the many challenges we face, the elimination of malnutrition is a possibility. It can be achieved in practical terms, if only we have the will to work together.

The Road to Good Nutrition presents a collective vision, and it is the product of a collective effort. As Editor-in-Chief of the volume, it has been my privilege to work with an international Editorial Board that has brought to the table the expertise of many different disciplines and the experience of many decades. For the generous provision of their time, their telling insights and their firm commitment to the creation of this book I would like to offer my warm thanks to Marc Van Ameringen, Hans Konrad Biesalski, Junshi Chen, Klaus Kraemer, Asma Lateef, Marie Ruel and Venkatesh Mannar. Klaus Kraemer and Marie Ruel worked tirelessly to ensure that the book's contents were as accurate and up-to-the-minute as possible; Hans Konrad Biesalski provided important new research in the field of hidden hunger; Asma Lateef gave perspectives on the growing role of civil society in combating malnutrition, and Marc Van Ameringen on the part that donor organizations can play; while Junshi Chen and Venkatesh Mannar offered the viewpoints derived from the experience of China and India respectively, helping to ensure that our perspective was as global as possible. I am grateful to all of them.

> *"Everyone has the right to a standard of living adequate for the health and well-being of himself and of his family, including food, clothing, housing and medical care and necessary social services, and the right to security in the event of unemployment, sickness, disability, widowhood, old age or other lack of livelihood in circumstances beyond his control."*
>
> **Universal Declaration of Human Rights:** *Article 25 (1948)*

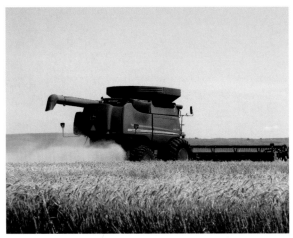

Nutrition-sensitive agricultural policies are essential to combat the global scourge of malnutrition
Sno Shuu Photography

> *"A hungry man can't see right or wrong. He just sees food."*
>
> **Pearl S. Buck** *(1892–1973)*

I am likewise grateful to the contributors who graciously provided the content for this book, taking time out of their packed agendas and busy traveling schedules to craft their individual chapters. My thanks go to Tom Arnold, Hans Konrad Biesalski, Martin Bloem, Joachim von Braun, Alan Dangour, Stuart Gillespie, John Hoddinott, Eileen Kennedy, Alain Labrique, Asma Lateef, Marguerite B. Lucea, Saskia de Pee, Victoria Quinn, Marie Ruel, Werner Schultink and Patrick Webb. They have each helped to shape this work, offering world-class thinking in response to a global challenge. My thanks, and the thanks of the entire Editorial Board, go to each of them.

Last but by absolutely no means least, I would like to thank David Nabarro for his foreword to this volume, whose sentiments I can only echo. I hope that it will help to spread the good news of SUN yet further and encourage yet more support for the Movement.

The road that leads us towards good nutrition is not a short one. Nor is it an easy one. But it is one that we can negotiate if we walk it together.

Manfred Eggersdorfer

SVP Nutrition Science and Advocacy, DSM

Kaiseraugst, June 2013

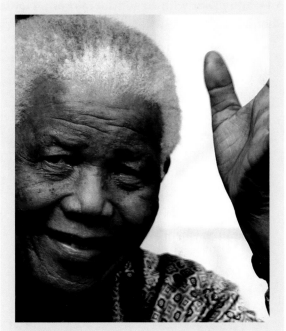

Nelson Mandela
Simon Dawson / AP

"Hunger is an aberration of the civilized world. It is the result of civil wars, oppressive governments, and famines of biblical proportions. Families are torn asunder by the question of who will eat. As global citizens, we must free children from the nightmare of poverty and abuse and deprivation. We must protect parents from the horrifying dilemma of choosing who will live. Hunger is a basic need that must be met before anyone can escape the depths of ignorance, before any society can stand without aid, but more importantly, before any child's body can survive the onslaught of disease such as the scourges of HIV, TB and malaria."

Nelson Mandela, 2004

V **A Healthy Diet with Essential Micronutrients is the Basis for a Healthy Life**

Poor diet is the 4th biggest global risk factor for disease.

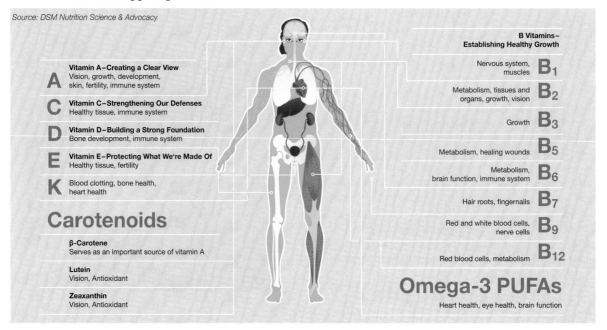

Life Expectancy Increasing (between 1990 and 2010)

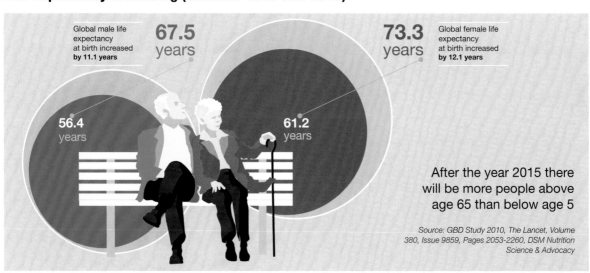

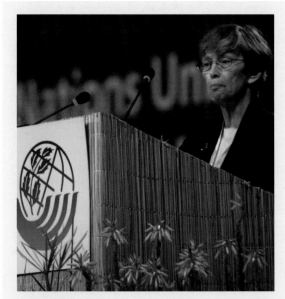

Carol Bellamy, UNICEF
Source: www.iisd.ca

"*Vitamin and mineral deficiency (VMD) touches the lives of perhaps a third of the world's people. After a decade of dramatic developments, the facts are known, the solutions are available, and the cause is one in which many individuals and organizations – governments, the private sector, the medical and scientific community, civil society – can all become involved. The challenge is therefore clear. And when so much could be achieved for so many and for so little, it would be a matter of global disgrace if vitamin and mineral deficiency were not brought under control in the years immediately ahead.*"

Carol Bellamy

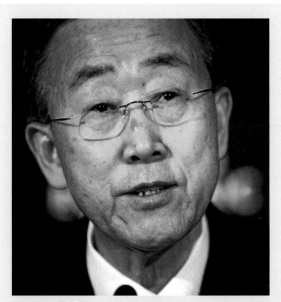

Ban Ki-moon, United Nations Secretary-General, during a press conference at the 2011 World Economic Forum in Davos, Switzerland
Source: WEF 2011

"*In our world of plenty, no one should live in hunger. No child should have his growth stunted by malnutrition. No child should have her opportunity for a better life curtailed even before she is born, because her mother was undernourished.*"

Ban Ki-moon, World Food Prize laureate award ceremony, 2012.

How to Use this Book

The Road to Good Nutrition presents a snapshot of current thinking about the world's contemporary nutrition challenges. Written with the general reader in mind, it examines the topic of nutrition from many angles, providing insights and opinions from some of the world's leading experts in the field and backing up their arguments with extensive graphical information and up-to-the-minute photographs.

As will be seen from the Executive Summary, this book presents a coherent set of arguments which may be read in sequential form from cover to cover, starting with an analysis of the hugely damaging effects of stunting and concluding with a call to concerted action in the here and now. Conversely, the book's chapters may be read individually, and in non-sequential order, by the reader wishing to focus on this or that specific aspect of the subject.

Each chapter follows approximately the same format, with key messages highlighted at the outset, a personal conclusion from the author, and a list of publications and websites for further study of the chapter topic. Graphics have been used from a wide variety of sources to interpret and enrich the flow of the narrative. These have been recreated in the house style of the book and their source acknowledged. Case studies, stories and thought pieces have likewise been quoted from a variety of sources and their original publication details provided. Where necessary in view of the constraints of space, these have been abridged, but they have not been otherwise re-edited or re-formulated. In presenting such a wide variety of graphic and written material to complement the main argumentation of the book, we hope to provide the general reader with an impression of the global nature of nutrition and of the need for multi-sectoral solutions worldwide. The Editorial Board gratefully acknowledges the use of all material drawn from the public realm and re-presented in this volume.

The book's individual chapters are supplemented by a list of key definitions and, in Chapter Thirteen, an overview of key scientific and policy milestones, plus a list of key organizations in the world of nutrition. The index will also help the reader to navigate around what is by any measure a complex and multi-faceted subject.

Given the global nature of nutrition and the rapid evolution of current thinking in this field, a book such as *The Road to Good Nutrition* can never be complete or comprehensive. It may, however, function as a guidebook for those wishing to find out more about this topic, and will hopefully encourage many readers to take an active part in this global journey themselves.

Contents

Key Definitions

Acute malnutrition (also known as wasting)
Reflects a recent and severe process that has led to substantial weight loss, usually associated with starvation and/or disease. Acute malnutrition is calculated by comparing the weight-for-height (WFH) of a child with a reference population of well-nourished and healthy children. Often used to assess the severity of emergencies because it is strongly related to mortality.[1]

Birthrate
The proportion of births in a defined population.

Blanket feeding
Feeding of all persons or households in an affected population without targeting specific individuals or subgroup.

Blanket supplementary feeding program
Nutrition programs that target a food supplement to all members of a specified at risk group, regardless of whether they have moderate acute malnutrition. Blanket supplementary feeding programs are usually implemented in combination with a general food distribution. They primarily aim to prevent deterioration in the nutritional status of at-risk groups.

BMI-for-age
A nutritional index based on anthropometry, used for the assessment of acute malnutrition in adolescents. It relates BMI (body mass index) to age in order to take into account changes in anthropometric measurements during puberty.[2]

Body mass index (BMI)
A nutritional index based on anthropometry, used for the assessment of acute malnutrition in adults. It is measured using body mass index or weight/height^2 (kg/m^2).[2]

Breast milk substitute (BMS)
Any food marketed or otherwise represented as a partial or total replacement for breast milk, whether or not suitable for that purpose.[1]

Chronic malnutrition
Chronic malnutrition, also known as stunting, is a sign of 'shortness' and develops over a long period of time. In children and adults, it is measured through the height-for-age nutritional index.[2]

Common results framework
Government ministries and other stakeholders in SUN countries are aligning their efforts to scale up nutrition using Common Results Frameworks (CRFs). These frameworks ensure that all share the same goals and implement effective and aligned actions to achieve these goals. Country CRFs include both specific nutrition interventions and nutrition-sensitive approaches to development.[1]

Community participation
The active involvement of the community in the planning, management, implementation, monitoring and evaluation of services and projects.[2]

Complementary feeding
The transition from exclusive breastfeeding to complementary feeding – typically covers the period from 6 to 24 months of age. This is a critical period of growth during which nutrient deficiencies and illnesses contribute globally to higher rates of undernutrition among children under five years of age. The SUN Movement aligns with the WHO recommendation that infants should be exclusively breastfed for the first six months of life to achieve optimal growth, development and health. Thereafter, infants should receive nutritionally adequate and safe complementary foods, while continuing to breastfeed for up to two years or more.[1]

Coverage
The proportion of the target population reached by an intervention. Coverage is a key indicator for monitoring and evaluating interventions.[2]

Crude mortality rate
The proportion of a defined population who die each day expressed over 10,000. This is the most useful indicator in determining the severity of an emergency situation.[2]

Dehydration
Excessive loss of body fluids.[2]

Diabetes
Type 1 diabetes, also sometimes called juvenile-onset diabetes or insulin-dependent diabetes is a chronic condition in which the pancreas produces little or no insulin.

Type 2 diabetes, also sometimes called adult-onset or non-insulin-dependent diabetes, is a chronic condition that affects the way the body metabolizes sugars. With type 2 diabetes, the body either resists the effects of insulin or else does not produce enough insulin.

"Diabesity" is a term coined by Dr Francine Kaufman to indicate a combination of diabetes and obesity.

Diarrhea
The presence of three or more loose or fluid stools over a 24-hour period, accompanied or not by blood, mucous or fever. Diarrhea is caused by various bacteria or by viruses, or may be a symptom of other infections. Diarrhea is one of the major killers of young children in developing countries and in emergencies.[2]

Double burden of malnutrition
The "double burden of malnutrition" is defined as the coexistence of undernutrition and overweight in the same community or even the same household.

Dry feeding
Food provided in the form of a dry (take-home) ration.[2]

Early warning system
An information system designed to monitor indicators that may predict or forewarn of impending food shortages or famine.[2]

Emergency school feeding
Food provided either as a cooked meal or supplement in school or as a take-home ration to improve school attendance and performance, and to alleviate hunger.[2]

Endemic disease
An infectious disease that occurs throughout the year in a population, such as malaria, worms or chest infections.[2]

Enrichment
When micronutrients lost or removed during food processing are added back or restored in the final product (e.g., wheat flour is enriched with vitamin B1, niacin and iron).[2]

Essential fatty acids (EFAs)
Fatty acids that cannot be constructed within an organism from other components by any known chemical pathways, and therefore must be obtained from food sources, such as flaxseed oil and sunflower oil.[2]

Exclusive breastfeeding
(adapted from WHO definition) Breast milk contains all the nutrients an infant needs in the first six months of life. It protects against common childhood diseases such as diarrhea and pneumonia, and may also have longer-term benefits such as lowering mean blood pressure and cholesterol, and reducing the prevalence of obesity and type-2 diabetes. The SUN Movement aligns with the WHO recommendation on exclusive breastfeeding whereby infants receive only breast milk, no other liquids or solids – not even water – for the first six months of life, to achieve optimal growth, development and health. Thereafter, infants should receive nutritionally adequate and safe complementary foods, while continuing to breastfeed for up to two years or more.[1]

Food access
Income or other resources are adequate to obtain sufficient and appropriate food through home production, buying, barter, gathering, etc. Food may be available but not accessible to people who do not have adequate land to cultivate or enough money to buy it.[2]

Food aid
In-kind rations of food, which can be sourced locally, regionally or internationally.[3]

Food assistance
The set of interventions designed to provide access to food to vulnerable and food insecure populations. Generally included are instruments like food transfers, vouchers and cash transfers to ensure access to food of a given quantity, quality or value.[3]

Food diversity
A diet containing a wide range of different types of foodstuffs, used as a measure of household food access.[2]

Food fortification
The process of adding micronutrients to foodstuffs, during or after processing, to bring micronutrient levels over and above amounts in the original food product.[2]

Food security
Food security exists when all people, at all times, have physical and economic access to sufficient safe and nutritious food that meets their dietary needs and food preferences for an active and healthy life.

Fortificant
The vitamins and minerals added to fortified foods.[2]

Fortified blended foods (FBFs)
A mixture of cereals and other ingredients (such as soya beans preferably de-hulled, pulses, oil seeds, dried skimmed milk, and possibly sugar) that has been milled, blended, pre-cooked by extrusion or roasting, and fortified with a pre-mix of adequate amount and with a wide range of vitamins and minerals. Fortified blended foods include Corn Soya Blend and Wheat Soy Blend.[2]

Growth reference
Nutritional indices are compared to expected anthropometric values for an individual of the same sex and age. A growth reference reflects the expected values in a reference population.[2]

5

Growth standard

Nutritional indices are compared to expected anthropometric values for an individual of the same sex and age. A growth standard is based on prescriptive criteria and involves value or normative judgments.[2]

Healthcare system

All organizations and institutions involved in the delivery of health services, including governmental, non-governmental, private organizations and institutions.[2]

Hidden hunger

Occurs when a population that may be consuming enough calories is not receiving enough micronutrients (vitamins and minerals), negatively impacting the health, cognitive development and economic development of over 2 billion people worldwide.[1]

Hunger

A weakened condition brought about by prolonged lack of food. Hunger can lead to malnutrition.[1]

Infant

A child less than 12 months old.[2]

Infant and young child feeding (IYCF)

Term used to describe the feeding of infants (less than 12 months old) and young children (12–23 months old). IYCF programs focus on the protection, promotion and support of exclusive breastfeeding for the first six months; timely introduction of complementary feeding and continued breastfeeding for two years or beyond.[1]

Infant formula

A breast milk substitute formulated industrially in accordance with applicable Codex Alimentarius standards to satisfy the normal nutritional requirements of infants up to six months of age.[2]

Information, education and communication (ICE)

Methods of providing people with an informed base for making choices. Nutrition information refers to knowledge, such as information about new foods that are being introduced in an emergency situation. Nutrition education refers to training or orientation for a particular purpose such as support for breastfeeding. Nutrition communication refers to the method by which information is imparted.[2]

Low birth weight

Weight at birth less than 2,500 grams.[1]

Macronutrients

Nutrients that humans consume in the largest quantities which provide bulk energy and are needed for a wide range of body functions and processes. The three macronutrients are fat, protein and carbohydrate.[2]

Malnutrition

A condition resulting when a person's diet does not provide adequate nutrients for growth and maintenance or if they are unable to fully utilize the food they eat due to illness.[1]

Micronutrient deficiency

A lack or shortage of a micronutrient, such as a vitamin or mineral, that is essential in small amounts for the proper growth and metabolism of a human or other living organism.[2]

Micronutrients

Essential vitamins and minerals required by the body throughout the lifecycle in miniscule amounts.[1]

Millennium Development Goals (MDGs)

At the Millennium Summit in September 2000 the largest gathering of world leaders in history adopted the UN Millennium Declaration, committing their nations to a new global partnership to reduce extreme poverty and setting out a series of time-bound targets, with a deadline of 2015, that have become known as the Millennium Development Goals. The Millennium Development Goals (MDGs) are quantified targets for addressing extreme poverty in its many dimensions – income poverty, hunger, disease, lack of adequate shelter, and exclusion – while promoting gender equality, education, and environmental sustainability. They are also basic human rights – the rights of each person on the planet to health, education, shelter, and security.[1]

Moderate acute malnutrition (MAM)

Acute malnutrition, also known as wasting, develops as a result of recent rapid weight loss or a failure to gain weight. The degree of acute malnutrition is classified as either moderate or severe. Moderate malnutrition is defined by a mid-upper arm circumference (MUAC) between 115 mm and <125 mm or a WFH between -3 z-score and <-2 z-score of the median (WHO standards) or WFH as a percentage of the median 70% and <80% ((National Center for Health Statistics [NCHS] references).[2]

Multi-stakeholder platform

A shared space for cross-sector stakeholders – including government representatives, civil society, UN agencies, donors, businesses and the research and technical community – to come together within a SUN country to align activities and take joint responsibility for scaling up nutrition, including setting shared targets and coordinated, costed plans of action.[1]

Non-communicable diseases (NCDs)

Non-communicable diseases (NCDs) – also known as chronic diseases – are not transmitted from person to person. NCDs can progress slowly and persist in the body for decades. The main types of NCDs include cardiovascular disease, cancers, respiratory diseases and diabetes.

Nutrition security

Achieved when secure access to an appropriately nutritious diet is coupled with a sanitary environment, adequate health services and care.[2] Nutrition security exists when, in addition to having access to a healthy and balanced diet, people also have access to adequate caregiving practices and to a safe and healthy environment that allows them to stay healthy and utilize the foods they eat effectively.

Nutritional status

The internal state of an individual as it relates to the availability and utilization of nutrients at the cellular level.[2]

Nutrition-sensitive approaches

Strategies and plans that address the underlying and basic causes of malnutrition and take into consideration the cross-sector impact of nutrition.[1]

Nutrition-specific interventions

Programs and plans that are designed to address the direct causes of malnutrition and to have a specific impact on nutrition outcomes. These include: support for exclusive breastfeeding; appropriate complementary feeding; micronutrient fortification and supplementation; and treatment of acute malnutrition.[1]

Nutrition-specific interventions and programs

Interventions or programs that address the underlying determinants of fetal and child nutrition and development – food security; adequate caregiving resources at the maternal, household and community levels; and access to health services and a safe and hygienic environment – and incorporate specific nutrition goals and actions. Nutrition-sensitive programs can serve as delivery platforms for nutrition-specific interventions, potentially increasing their scale, coverage, and effectiveness. Examples: agriculture and food security; social safety nets; early child development; maternal mental health; women's empowerment; child protection; schooling; water, sanitation, and hygiene; health and family planning services.[4]

Obesity

Obesity for adults is a BMI 30 to 39.99.
Morbidly obese for adults is BMI of 40 or greater.

Overweight

Overweight for adults is a BMI between 25 and 29.00.

Ready-to-use foods (RUF)

RUF can be eaten without further preparation or cooking. Most RUF have very low moisture content and so can be stored without refrigeration. They are typically energy-dense, mineral- and vitamin-fortified foods and can be used for the treatment or prevention of various types of undernutrition.[2]

Ready-to-use supplementary foods (RUSF)

Energy-dense, mineral- and vitamin-fortified foods that are designed to provide the quantities of macro- and micronutrients needed for the treatment or prevention of moderate acute malnutrition. RUSFs can be eaten without further preparation or cooking and are given as a supplement to the ordinary diet. They have very low moisture content and so can be stored without refrigeration.[2]

Ready-to-use therapeutic foods (RUTF)

Specialized ready-to-eat, portable, shelf-stable products, available as pastes, spreads or biscuits, that are used in a prescribed manner to treat children with severe acute malnutrition.[1]

Recommended daily allowance (RDA)

The average daily dietary intake level that is sufficient to meet the nutrient requirements of nearly all (approximately 98 percent) healthy individuals.[2]

School feeding

Provision of meals or snacks to schoolchildren to improve nutrition and promote education.[2]

Selective feeding programs

Targeted supplementary feeding or therapeutic care programs that admit individuals based on anthropometric, clinical or social criteria for correction of acute malnutrition.[2]

Severe acute malnutrition (SAM)

Acute malnutrition, also known as wasting, develops as a result of recent rapid weight loss or a failure to gain weight. The degree of acute malnutrition is classified as either moderate or severe. A child with severe acute malnutrition is highly vulnerable and has a high mortality risk. Severe acute malnutrition is defined by the presence of bilateral pitting oedema or severe wasting, defined by MUAC <115 mm or a WFH <-3 z-score (WHO standards) or WFH <70% of the median (NCHS references)).[2]

7

Stunting

Low height-for-age measurement used as an indicator of chronic malnutrition, calculated by comparing the height-for-age of a child with a reference population of well-nourished and healthy children.[1]

SUN donor convener

A representative from a donor organization in each SUN county who is: actively engaged in the country, involved in financially supporting nutrition-specific and/or nutrition-sensitive programs and committed to increasing resources for nutrition.[1]

SUN government Focal Point

A high-level individual appointed in each SUN country to play a critical role in leading coordination efforts for catalyzing efforts to advance nutrition in their country. Focal Points help to establish the multi-stakeholder platforms that strengthen coordination to improve support for national plans. They work across sectors and bring ministries and government departments together with local development partners, civil society organizations, businesses and UN agencies.[1]

SUN Multi-Partner Trust Fund (MPTF)

A fund established in March 2012 by participating UN agencies and contributing partners to provide catalytic grants to governments, UN agencies, civil society groups, other SUN stakeholders to facilitate the development and implementation of government or stakeholder actions for scaling up nutrition.[1]

Supplementary feeding

The provision of food to the nutritionally or socially vulnerable in addition to the general food distribution to treat or prevent malnutrition.[2]

Supplementary feeding program

Nutrition programs that aim to prevent individuals with moderate acute malnutrition from developing severe acute malnutrition, to treat those with moderate acute malnutrition and to prevent the development of moderate malnutrition in individuals. Supplementary feeding programs can be blanket or targeted.[2]

Supplementation

Provision of nutrients either via a food or as a tablet, capsule, syrup, or powder to boost the nutritional content of the diet.

Sustainable development goals

One of the main outcomes of the Rio+20 Conference was the agreement by member states to launch a process to develop a set of sustainable development goals (SDGs), which will build upon the Millennium Development Goals and converge with the post-2015 development agenda. It was decided to establish an "*inclusive and transparent intergovernmental process open to all stakeholders, with a view to developing global sustainable development goals to be agreed by the General Assembly*".

In the Rio+20 outcome document, member States agreed that sustainable development goals (SDGs) must:

1. Be based on Agenda 21 and the Johannesburg Plan of Implementation.

2. Fully respect all the Rio Principles.

3. Be consistent with international law.

4. Build upon commitments already made.

5. Contribute to the full implementation of the outcomes of all major summits in the economic, social and environmental fields.

6. Focus on priority areas for the achievement of sustainable development, being guided by the outcome document.

7. Address and incorporate in a balanced way all three dimensions of sustainable development and their interlinkages.

8. Be coherent with and integrated into the United Nations development agenda beyond 2015.

9. Not divert focus or effort from the achievement of the Millennium Development Goals.

10. Include active involvement of all relevant stakeholders, as appropriate, in the process.

It was further agreed that SDGs must be:

- Action-oriented

- Concise

- Easy to communicate

- Limited in number

- Aspirational

- Global in nature

- Universally applicable to all countries while taking into account different national realities, capacities and levels of development and respecting national policies and priorities.

The outcome document further specifies that the development of SDGs should:

- Be useful for pursuing focused and coherent action on sustainable development

- Contribute to the achievement of sustainable development

- Serve as a driver for implementation and mainstreaming of sustainable development in the UN system as a whole

- Address and be focused on priority areas for the achievement of sustainable development

The Rio+20 outcome document *The Future We Want* resolved to establish an inclusive and transparent intergovernmental process on SDGs that is open to all stakeholders with a view to developing global sustainable development goals to be agreed by the UN General Assembly. The outcome document mandated the creation of an inter-governmental Open Working Group, that will submit a report to the 68th session of the General Assembly containing a proposal for sustainable development goals for consideration and appropriate action. The outcome document specifies that the process leading to the SDGs needs to be coordinated and coherent with the processes considering the post-2015 development agenda and that initial input to the work of the Open Working Group will be provided by the UN Secretary-General in consultation with national governments.[5]

Targeted supplementary feeding program

Nutrition programs that provide nutritional support to individuals with moderate acute malnutrition. They generally target children under five, malnourished pregnant and breastfeeding mothers, and other nutritionally at-risk individuals in the presence of a general food distribution. The objectives are primarily curative and aim to rehabilitate individuals with moderate acute malnutrition, prevent individuals with moderate acute malnutrition from developing severe acute malnutrition, prevent malnutrition in at-risk individuals and rehabilitate referrals from the treatment of severe acute malnutrition.[2]

UN REACH (Renewed Effort Against Child Hunger and Undernutrition)

Established in 2008 by the Food and Agricultural Organization (FAO), the United Nations Children's Fund (UNICEF), the World Food Program (WFP), and the World Health Organization (WHO) to assist governments of countries with a high burden of child and maternal undernutrition to accelerate the scale-up of food and nutrition actions. The International Fund for Agricultural Development (IFAD) joined REACH later on with an advisory role. REACH operates at country level as a facilitating mechanism in the coordination of UN and other partners' support to national nutrition scale-up plans.[1]

Undernutrition

An insufficient intake of energy, protein or micronutrients, that in turn leads to nutritional deficiency. Undernutrition encompasses stunting, wasting and micronutrient deficiencies.[2]

Underweight

Wasting or stunting or a combination of both, defined by weight-for-age below the -2 z-score line. [2]

Vulnerability

The characteristics of a person or group in terms of their capacity to anticipate, cope with, resist and recover from the impact of a natural (or human-made) hazard.[2]

Wasting (also known as acute malnutrition)

Reflects a recent and severe process that has led to substantial weight loss, usually associated with starvation and/or disease. Wasting is calculated by comparing the weight-for-height of a child with a reference population of well-nourished and healthy children. Often used to assess the severity of emergencies because it is strongly related to mortality.[1]

Weight-for-length/height or BMI-for-age below the -2 z-score line. Severely wasted is below the -3 z-score line.[2]

Z-score

An indicator of how far a measurement is from the median, also known as a standard deviation (SD) score. The reference lines on the growth charts (labeled 1, 2, 3, -1, -2, -3) are called z-score lines; they indicate how far points are above or below the median z-score = 0).[2]

This glossary draws on a variety of sources. The provenance of individual definitions is indicated by a reference as follows:

1 UNICEF SUN 2012
2 UNICEF Training on Nutrition in Emergencies, Glossary of Terms
3 Omamo SW, Gentilini U, Sandström S (eds). Revolution: From food aid to food assistance. Innovations in overcoming hunger. 2010. WfP, Rome, Italy.
4 The Lancet 2013 Series on Maternal and Child Nutrition, adapted from Scaling Up Nutrition and Shekar and colleagues, 2013
5 United Nations Sustainable Development Knowledge Platform, June 2013

Executive Summary

Since 2008 many governments, civil society organizations, research groups and intergovernmental agencies have sought ways to scale up effective actions for better nutrition. The collective experience to date suggests that such efforts are successful if all the different groups that seek to enable improvements in people's nutrition work *together* in support of sound national policies, the implementation of effective interventions, and sector programs that are sensitive to the determinants of malnutrition. *The Road to Good Nutrition* brings together the thinking of many world experts on this subject, each of whom addresses from their specialist perspective the question of how to improve the nutritional status of the world's population as a whole.

Chapter One, by Martin Bloem (Chief Nutrition and HIV/AIDS Policy/Global Coordinator UNAIDS – United Nations World Food Program; Adjunct Associate Professor, – Johns Hopkins Bloomberg School of Public Health, Baltimore, USA) explains how stunting is the result of inadequate nutrition in early life and how it has severe consequences that last a lifetime. Stunting prevents individuals from achieving their potential, physically, intellectually and economically. Its consequences are severe and irreparable, both for the individual and for society as a whole. While the world has seen significant advances in the field of nutrition since the development of the Millennium Development Goals (MDGs), which were to be reached by 2015, stunting remains a problem of global dimensions: according to the latest report of UNICEF/WHO/World Bank (2012), 165 million children under 5 are stunted, and many school-age children, adolescents and adults today suffer the consequences of the stunting that they experienced during their early years of life. Chapter One outlines the problem of stunting and traces it to inadequate nutrition, especially in the first 1,000 days of life. It argues that the right to adequate nutrition (as opposed to simply food) should be recognized as a Human Right.

Chapter Two, by Marie Ruel (Director, Poverty, Health and Nutrition Division, International Food Policy Research Institute [IFPRI], Washington DC, USA) explains that food security and nutrition security are related but distinct concepts. Infants, young children, pregnant and breastfeeding women are especially vulnerable to undernutrition. For this reason, nutrition interventions must focus on the critical 'first 1,000 days' window of opportunity. Marie Ruel explains how achieving food and nutrition security is a multi-faceted challenge which requires a multi-sectoral approach – a theme which reappears in various forms throughout this book.

Food security is necessary, but not sufficient, to ensure nutrition and to prevent childhood malnutrition. Children also need their caregivers to provide them with appropriate feeding, caregiving, hygiene, and health-seeking practices in order to grow, develop and stay healthy. Food systems can play a critical role in protecting both food security and nutrition if careful attention is paid to targeting the poor, reducing inequalities, including gender inequalities, and incorporating nutrition goals and action where relevant.

The book's third chapter is authored by Hans Konrad Biesalski, Head of Department, Biological Chemistry and Nutrition, University of Hohenheim , Managing Director of the Food Security Center in Stuttgart, Germany. Drawing on Hans Konrad Biesalski's recently published work *Hidden Hunger* (Springer Verlag 2012) this chapter describes the phenomenon of hidden hunger. This term refers to a chronic lack of vitamins and minerals, which is not immediately apparent and which can exist for a long time before clinical signs of malnutrition become obvious. It affects over 3 billion people worldwide, contributing to many millions of deaths especially in children and young females, and also increasing the risk of non-communicable diseases such as diabetes, cardiovascular disease, cancer and osteoporosis. Linked to a general decline in meeting nutritional standards, hidden hunger is also a problem in the developed world. Solutions are nevertheless available: many countries have implemented mandatory or voluntary fortification of folic acid, vitamin D or iodine. The experience of many countries indicates that the fortification of staple or processed foods may be an efficient way to provide an adequate intake of micronutrients.

Eileen Kennedy (Professor of Nutrition and Former Dean of the Friedman School of Nutrition Science and Policy at Tufts University, Boston, USA) authors Chapter Four, which deals with the recent phenomenon of obesity. The current increase in obesity in the global population is unprecedented: Worldwide, approximately 1.4 billion adults are overweight, and 500 million are obese. This phenomenon is closely linked to inadequate nutrition, and is driving a massive increase in the incidence of nutrition and lifestyle-related non-communicable diseases (NCDs). This rise in NCDs is placing an increasing burden on social and healthcare systems. The challenge is daunting. Eileen Kennedy argues that the international community must aggressively implement multi-pronged strategies to combat overweight and obesity, while at the same time tackling undernutrition.

John Hoddinott, Deputy Director, Poverty Health and Nutrition Division, IFPRI, Washington DC, USA, presents Chapter Five, whose subject is the economic cost of malnutrition. In addition to its substantial human costs, undernutrition has lifelong economic consequences. John Hoddinott argues, however, that there exist feasible solutions to many dimensions of undernutrition, and that fighting undernutrition has considerable economic benefits – most notably in terms of improving schooling, cognitive skills and economic productivity. Spending that reduces both chronic undernutrition and micronutrient deficiencies is an excellent investment in economic terms, and is one of the smartest ways to spend global aid dollars.

John Hoddinott's economic analysis of the problem of malnutrition is followed by a presentation of best practice in nutrition by Victoria Quinn, who is Senior Vice President of Programs, Helen Keller International, New York, USA, and Adjunct Associate Professor, Friedman School of Nutrition Science and Policy, Boston, USA. Explaining that undernutrition is a complex and multifaceted phenomenon, and that it does not have a single cause, or a single solution, Victoria Quinn uses the Conceptual Framework of Young Child Nutrition to explain the causes of undernutrition and outline possible modes of intervention. At the national level, increased government investment in proven nutrition-specific and nutrition-sensitive interventions is essential for improving nutrition, while at the family level, women have a critical role to play.

Victoria Quinn's analysis of best practice in nutrition is complemented by a contribution from Werner Schultink, Associate Director, Nutrition Section, Programme Division, UNICEF, New York, on How to Improve Nutrition Through Effective Programming. Werner Schultink concludes that efforts to scale up nutrition programs are working, benefiting women and children and their communities in many countries, and points out that such programs all have common elements: political commitment, national policies and programs based on sound evidence and analysis, the presence of trained and skilled community workers collaborating with communities, effective communication and advocacy, and multisectoral, integrated service delivery.

Chapter Eight is penned by Joachim von Braun, Director of the Center for Development Research (ZEF) and Professor for Economic and Technological Change at the University of Bonn, Germany. Food prices today are not only set by supply and demand but also influenced by financial markets. Joachim von Braun explains how sudden price rises, or 'spikes', cause big problems for nutrition of the poor. He argues that healthy diets need to be affordable, which requires increased productivity in the food system to prevent high prices. Unfortunately poor countries are hit worst by spikes in food prices, as they cannot afford

adjustment measures. The solution therefore needs to be worked on globally, and the issue taken more seriously.

Joachim von Braun's price-specific analysis is followed by a broader interrogation of the governance of nutrition by Stuart Gillespie, Senior Research Fellow, Poverty, Health and Nutrition Division, IFPRI, and CEO of the Transform Nutrition Research Program Consortium. Taking the theme of Making Nutrition Good Politics, Stuart Gillespie outlines the potential of governance for improving the nutritional status of the world's poorest and most disadvantaged populations. Believing that progress in reducing undernutrition cannot be sustained where governance systems are weak or absent, he reasons that strong leadership – in the form of ambassadors championing the political cause, as well as more mid-level, lateral leadership to facilitate intersectoral action – is fundamental to success.

While Stuart Gillespie focuses on governance as one of the factors essential for delivering improved nutrition, Tom Arnold (Member of Lead Group of the Scaling Up Nutrition [SUN] movement and former CEO of Concern Worldwide) explains the key role that advocacy has to play. Noting that it requires a solid evidential base in order to succeed, Tom Arnold outlines the importance of presenting arguments in simple and powerful language and of maintaining commitment and momentum over time in order to bring about change. An important political and policy mechanism for achieving progress is the SUN Movement, which brings together governments, civil society and the private sector to work in a coordinated way to reduce early childhood undernutrition. Real progress can be made over the next decade if we deliver on what we know is possible, concludes Tom Arnold.

The following chapter of this book, number Eleven, is unique in being co-written by three authors: Alan Dangour (Senior Lecturer, London School of Hygiene and Tropical Medicine [LSHTM]; Marguerite B Lucea (Faculty Research Associate, Johns Hopkins University School of Nursing (JHUSON), Baltimore, MD; and Alain Labrique (Director, JHU Global mHealth Initiative and Assistant Professor, Department of International Health & Dept of Epidemiology (jt) Bloomberg School of Public Health). Together they present the power of innovation in the battle against malnutrition. In a chapter packed with topical case studies of innovation in practice, they argue that innovations across the entire span of human nutrition have for centuries targeted aspects of the farm-to-table continuum, and show how recent transformative innovations targeting distribution systems, leveraging public-private partnerships, and utilizing technological advances have the potential to catalyze research and improve nutrition in both the developed and developing world.

Asma Lateef, Director, Bread for the World Institute, Washington DC, USA, follows with a chapter on the role that civil society has to play in improving nutrition. Describing hunger and malnutrition as an 'unfinished agenda', Asma Lateef argues that food security and nutrition should be explicitly addressed in the goals for the post-2015 development framework, and that stunting should be a priority indicator. Civil society organizations are uniquely positioned to advocate for greater attention to hunger and malnutrition, and can play an important role in elevating nutrition as a priority for the next set of goals. She concludes that communicating the fundamental role that good nutrition has to play during pregnancy and early childhood must be part of advocacy efforts in the near future.

The final chapter of the book is written by Saskia de Pee (Adjunct assistant Professor Friedman School of Nutrition Science and Policy, Tufts University, Boston, and visiting assistant Professor, Wageningen University, the Netherlands). Saskia de Pee's contribution describes how the world of nutrition has evolved in recent decades. Throughout the 20th century, knowledge and approaches for addressing malnutrition developed within specific scientific and professional disciplines, but there was limited cross-disciplinary coordination, even with other players in

the food and health systems. Understanding the forms and consequences of undernutrition, being able to cost the economic impact of undernutrition, and having examples of what is required and what works to prevent undernutrition, including good governance, has generated the strong momentum behind nutrition that exists today. The involvement of so many is essential, and while everyone should focus on what they are good at, Saskia de Pee argues, there is a great deal of cross-disciplinary work to be done in a target-oriented manner. It is important to develop context-specific solutions based on the global body of knowledge and expertise, and to monitor, evaluate and share these experiences using the information and communication technology available today.

Finally Patrick Webb, Dean for Academic Affairs, Friedman School of Nutrition Science and Policy, Tufts University, Boston, USA, provides an eloquent afterword to this volume. "This book," he writes, "captures the fact that there has not been a time in recent decades when so many people agreed on what needs to be done or why. The momentum has to be maintained. The next decade of the 21st century should be focused squarely on a global effort to get it done well, while documenting how. Unless coherent, cost-effective actions with measurable impacts quickly emerge from the current cresting wave of goodwill toward nutrition, the wait for another may be far too long. Now is the time."

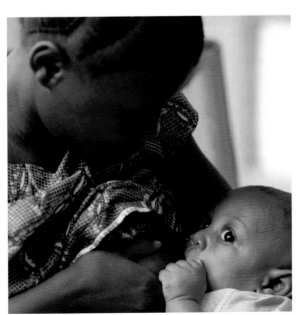

A well-nourished mother and infant: Elizabeth Farma 16, breastfeeds her two-month-old son Emmanuel at the Bonthe District Hospital, Sierra Leone
Source: UNICEF/NYHQ 2010-0952/Olivier Asselin

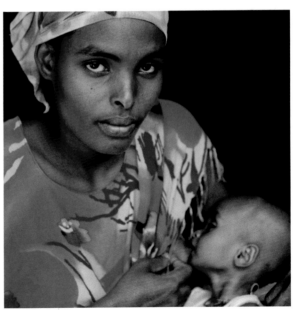

Malnourished mother breastfeeding her newborn in Kenya: the signs of malnourishment are evident in both mother and child
Source: Mike Bloem Photography

Maternal undernutrition – a mother's story (Bangladesh)

Farida is a Bangladeshi housewife of 23. She lives in the Sreepur Upazila, a rural subdistrict close to the capital, Dhaka. Married at the age of 17, within a year she fell pregnant. During her pregnancy, Farida had no access to skilled prenatal care or education. To stay healthy and aid her pregnancy she wore a *tabij* (a charm amulet) and drank *paani puri* (a mint drink). Unfortunately, after going into premature labor she lost her baby within half an hour of delivery. Two years later, Farida became pregnant once more, but received limited medical attention. Tragically her second child arrived stillborn.

Several months later, Farida met a Community Nutrition Worker from Plan Bangladesh's affiliate Prankteek, called Nurunnahar. She advised Farida to attend Plan's notional information sessions. At these sessions she learnt the importance of prenatal care, a nutritious diet and receiving proper rest during pregnancy. The lessons learned in the nutrition sessions were complemented by regular household visits from Nurunnahar, during which Farida could consult with her on questions or concerns.

When Farida became pregnant for a third time, she went to medical centers near her home for regular prenatal visits. On this occasion, she gave birth to a healthy baby boy. She breastfed him after delivery, and continued exclusive breastfeeding until her son was six months old. Now 17 months old, Farida's son is happy, healthy and keeps her very busy! Farida is thankful for her son, and wants others to be able to have the same opportunities for care that she did. "I have lost my first two children through ignorance," she said. "I don't want any other mother to have the same experience. I am grateful to Nurunnahar."

Source: Thousand Days Partnership, USA
http://thousanddays.org/success-story/material-undernutrition-a-mothers-story June 2011 (abridged)

The One Thousand Days Mission

The 1,000 days between a woman's pregnancy and her child's 2nd birthday offer a unique window of opportunity to shape healthier and more prosperous futures. The right nutrition during this 1,000-day window can have a profound impact on a child's ability to grow, learn, and rise out of poverty. It can also shape a society's long-term health, stability and prosperity.

Today, undernutrition is still a leading cause of death of young children throughout the world. For infants and children under the age of two, the consequences of undernutrition are particularly severe, often irreversible, and reach far into the future.

During pregnancy, undernutrition can have a devastating impact on the healthy growth and development of a child. Babies who are malnourished in the womb have a higher risk of dying in infancy and are more likely to face lifelong cognitive and physical deficits and chronic health problems.

For children under the age of two, undernutrition can be life threatening. It can weaken a child's immune system and make him or her more susceptible to dying from common illnesses such as pneumonia, diarrhea and malaria.

Source: Thousand Days Partnership, USA
http://thousanddays.org/about/

One Thousand Days Organization

Solutions to prevent and treat undernutrition already exist. Every day, 1,000 Days partners are putting proven solutions into action in communities around the world. By working in alignment with the Scaling Up Nutrition (SUN) Framework, 1,000 Days partners join a movement to work across sectors and specialties to achieve better nutrition results. By prioritizing proven nutrition solutions, progress is being made and lives are being changed for the better. Strong nutrition programs, sound policies and better investments can make a difference in the lives of mothers and children today in a way that dramatically improves the health and well-being of future generations of individuals, families and communities.

Source: Thousand Days Partnership, USA
http://thousanddays.org/resources/success-stories/

Chapter One

Preventing Stunting: Why it Matters, What it Takes

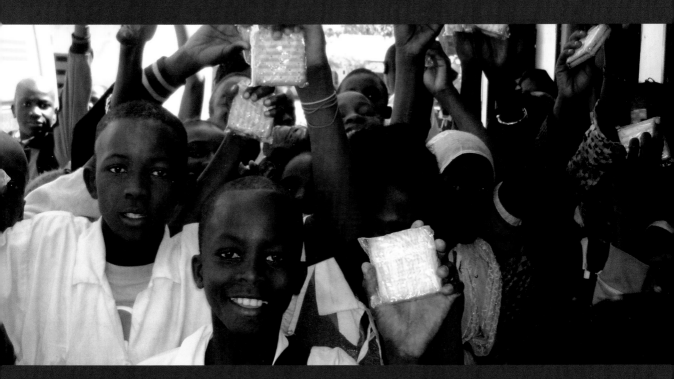

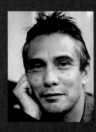

Martin Bloem
Senior Nutritionist and WFP's Global Coordinator UNAIDS – United Nations World Food Program; Adjunct Associate Professor, – Johns Hopkins Bloomberg School of Public Health, Baltimore, USA; Adjunct Associate Professor, – Friedman School of Nutrition Science and Policy, Tufts University, Boston, USA

"Hunger is not only a physical condition. It is a drain on economic development, a threat to global security, a barrier to health and education reform, and a trap for the millions of people worldwide who work from sun-up to sun-down every day to produce a harvest that often doesn't meet their needs... We have the resources to give every person in the world the tools they need to feed themselves and their children. So the question is not whether we can end hunger. It's whether we will."

Hillary Clinton, 2009

Key messages

- Stunting is the result of inadequate nutrition in early life and has severe consequences that last a lifetime.

- Stunting prevents individuals from achieving their potential, physically, intellectually and economically.

- Stunting affects not only individuals but also the entire societies to which they belong.

- The right to adequate nutrition should be recognized as a Human Right.

Recent improvements in nutrition

The world has seen significant developments in the field of nutrition since the development of the Millennium Development Goals (MDGs), which were to be reached by 2015, and included ending hunger and reducing underweight as part of MDG number 1.

In 2008, the Lancet published the first landmark series on nutrition, which summarized the magnitude and consequences of the nutrition problem, as well as a number of proven and low-cost solutions. In 2013, the follow-up series on the subject was published. Four critical points made by these two Lancet series are:

i) chronic undernutrition, or stunting, is considered the main nutrition problem because it is a key obstacle for development;

ii) the window to prevent stunting is very small: from conception to two years of age;

iii) stunting at two years of age is associated with ill health, poorer school performance, and an increased risk of obesity, diabetes, and other chronic diseases later in life; and

iv) economic analyses indicate the negative effects of poor nutrition in early life on the overall economic development of nations.

A stunted child at the age of two is deprived from achieving its full potential for the rest of his/her life, which is an enormous drain on the world's human resources. Sufficient knowledge exists about effective strategies for prevention, and these strategies should be implemented by all parties concerned.

Prevention of stunting is central to the Scaling Up Nutrition (SUN) movement, and there is wide recognition that the prevention of stunting should also feature prominently in the post-2015 development agenda.

According to the latest report of UNICEF/WHO/World Bank (2012), 165 million children under 5 are stunted, and many school-age children, adolescents and adults today suffer the consequences of the stunting that they experienced during their early years of life.

`15`

What 'stunting' indicates

Stunting is defined as inadequate linear growth, and this is due to the fact that nutrient intake does not meet nutrient needs. Furthermore, nutrient needs may be increased by illness, and illness also reduces appetite and interferes with nutrient utilization, thus increasing the difficulty of meeting nutrient needs with existing nutrient intakes. Stunting is a relatively easy indicator to measure, and reflects undernutrition during a critical period of development, in particular from conception until two years of age (i.e., the first 1,000 days of life). Inadequate nutrition during this period has severe consequences for life, because many developmental processes occur only during certain stages of life, and cannot (re)occur later in life.

Stunting develops during life *in utero* and the first two years after birth. It is a process of suboptimal growth and development that gradually accumulates to such an extent that body length is below that of 97.7 percent of children in the reference population. Children born with a low birth weight (<2500 g) due to restricted intrauterine growth are at great risk of remaining stunted. Beyond 24 months of age, stunting prevalence may still increase, but at a much slower pace.

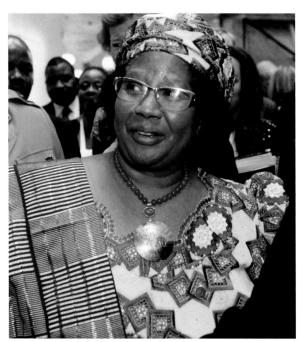

Malawi president Joyce Banda at the Nutrition for Growth conference in London, June 8, 2013
Soucre: Marisol Grandon/Department for International Development

Consequences of stunting

Lack of adequate nutrients in the first 1,000 days will, for example, lead to irreversible gaps in brain development. The outcome of brain development by the age of two years determines to a large extent a person's mental capacity for the rest of his/her life, including success in schooling and income earning.

Not only stunted children are affected by undernutrition: non-stunted children in populations with a considerable prevalence of stunting are also likely to be affected, i.e., they have not reached their full potential either, although their length is not below the cut-off which classifies them as 'stunted'.

Girls who grow up stunted are more likely to suffer complications during childbirth as adolescents or adults, because they have a smaller pelvis. Breaking the intergenerational cycle of undernutrition thus also requires good obstetric care, to facilitate the birth of a larger baby, born to a mother who may have been stunted herself but then had good nutrition pre-pregnancy and during pregnancy, resulting in the development of a larger infant in the womb.

Stunting typically co-occurs with micronutrient deficiencies, because foods that are rich in nutrients that are essential for linear growth are also good sources of other micronutrients. This also explains why stunting is such an important

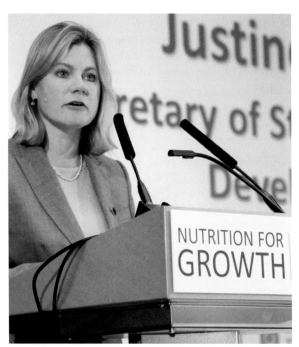

United Kingdom Secretary of State for International Development Justine Greening concludes the successful Nutrition for Growth conference, where world leaders gathered with businesses, scientific and civil society groups, committing to a historic reduction in undernutrition.
Soucre: Marisol Grandon/DfID

indicator, reflecting a shortage of essential nutrients during the most critical developmental phase in life.

As such, stunting has been linked to increased morbidity and mortality, delayed mental development, poor school performance, and reduced intellectual capacity. This in turn affects income in adult life, as well as economic productivity at national level. Furthermore, stunting is also related to increased risk of overweight and non-communicable disease such as diabetes and cardiovascular disease later in life.

The fact that much of this damage cannot be undone later in life means that it is essential to prevent stunting.

Prevention of stunting requires a nutritious diet

The prevention of undernutrition, or stunting, should start early in life, with interventions among at-risk populations that ensure that pregnant and lactating mothers are adequately nourished, that children receive exclusive breastfeeding during the first 6 months of life, and provision of adequate complementary feeding in addition to breastfeeding for children aged 6–23 months. Ensuring that pregnant women are adequately nourished may require intervening before pregnancy, i.e., during adolescence and before a next pregnancy, also because the impact of undernutrition already starts at conception.

The ultimate aim of interventions to prevent stunting should be that nutrient requirements of the individual child, also during life in utero, are met and that illness is prevented.

An individual needs approximately 40 different nutrients, in different amounts, in order to grow, develop and remain healthy. Meeting these requirements requires consumption of an adequately diverse diet, including breast milk, and a variety of plant-source foods (vegetables, fruits, staples), animal-source foods (dairy, eggs, fish, meat) as well as fortified foods. Where such a variety of foods is not available, or for those who (usually for economic reasons) cannot access such a variety, specially formulated foods may be required that fill the so-called 'nutrient gap'. These may need to be made available at lower than normal or no cost.

A home-fortification approach, where a small amount of a powder or lipid-based spread (<20 g, <100 kcal/d) is added to home-prepared foods, which adds vitamins, minerals and some other essential nutrients that are unlikely to be available in adequate amounts in the prevailing diet, is a promising strategy for preventing stunting, because it hardly changes the local diet and food practices. Another good option, which may be more familiar to families, is the introduction of specially formulated complementary foods, such as infant porridges that have a good content of essential nutrients.

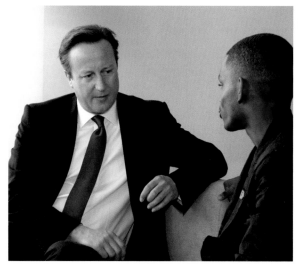

Tanzanian campaigner Frank shares his experience of hunger with British Prime Minister David Cameron at the Nutrition for Growth Summit
Source: Simon Davis/Department for International Development

Sun by the numbers

Scaling Up
NUTRITION

41 countries commited to Scaling Up Nutrition

Bangladesh	Guinea	Niger
Benin	Haiti	Nigeria
Burkina Faso	Indonesia	Pakistan
Burundi	Kenya	Peru
Cameroon	Kyrgyz Republic	Rwanda
Chad	Lao PDR	Senegal
Cote d'Ivoire	Madagascar	Sierra Leone
Democratic	Malawi	South Sudan
Republic of Congo	Mali	Sri Lanka
El Salvador	Mauritania	Tanzania
Ethiopia	Mozambique	Uganda
Gambia	Myanmar	Yemen
Ghana	Namibia	Zambia
Guatemala	Nepal	Zimbabwe

Which means the potential to reach **80** million children

By focusing on the critical **1,000** day window of opportunity to improve nutrition

There are **100+** committed partners accountable for supporting national plans

All working together to drive **1** global movement and unleash the potential of **milllions** of healthier, smarter and stronger children

Status: June 2013. Please see the SUN website for more recent updates.

17

Starting at stunting's basic cause, poverty and inequity

Both dietary diversity, which determines nutrient intake, and disease, which affects nutrient utilization and nutrient needs, and also food intake, are strongly linked to poverty. Stunting at the age of two years is therefore a reflection of inequity and also perpetuates this, due to its long-term negative health, economic, and social consequences for the individual, their offspring and the population they live in. Extreme poverty is the most critical problem the world has to cope with.

The first millennium development goal (MDG), which was formulated in 2000, set two indicators for reducing hunger: the number of undernourished people (energy intake not meeting requirements – based on food availability at national level and estimates of the population's energy needs) and the percentage of underweight children under five. Underweight, or too low weight-for-age, reflects both stunting as well as wasting, which are two different forms of undernutrition, in terms of immediate causes and possible solutions, and are therefore better recognized separately.

Since the 2008 and 2013 Lancet series identified stunting as the most critical indicator for malnutrition and the 65th

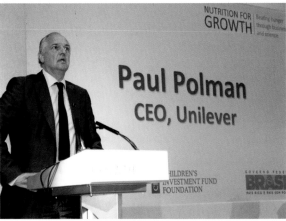

Paul Polman makes a heartfelt address to the assembled guests at the Nutrition for Growth conference, held in the Unilever building in central London, June 8, 2013
Soucre: Marisol Grandon/Department for International Development

World Health Assembly in 2012 set 6 global targets for nutrition, including as its first goal a 40 percent reduction of the global number of children under five who are stunted, there is a strong push among many stakeholders to include stunting as a target in the post-2015 development agenda (successor of the MDGs).

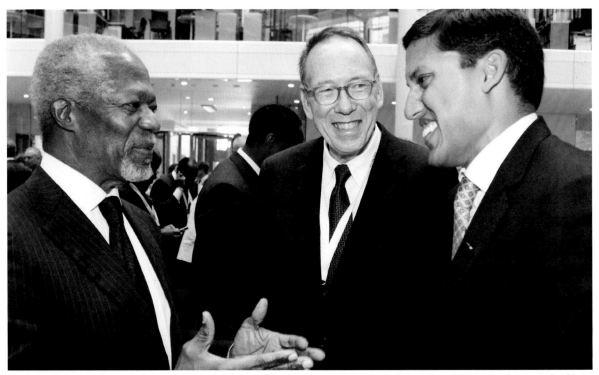

Former UN Secretary-General Kofi Annan and chairman of the Alliance for a Green Revolution in Africa talks to USAID administrator Dr Raj Shah at the conclusion of the Nutrition for Growth conference in London, 8 June, 2013
Soucre: Marisol Grandon/Department for International Development

Prevention of stunting should be a human right

Although child undernutriton has long been used as an indicator or proxy for poverty, the world has never united behind making prevention of undernutrition a goal in itself. As stunting is now recognized as so detrimental to development, depriving individuals of the possibility of having equal chances for the rest of their life, the prevention of undernutrition, or stunting, should be recognized as a human right. In view of the fact that it has such widespread consequences, impacting on so many aspects of life, it should not be regarded as merely a 'nutrition problem' that nutritionists should solve.

While nutrition has been mentioned as a component of the "right to food", "right to health" and "Convention on the Rights of the Child", the prevention of chronic undernutrition has not yet been recognized as a right. In fact, nutrition is mentioned sparsely in the various 'human rights' documents, which is apparently due to the fact that nutrition is not regarded as a right in itself but as an element of health or an outcome of lack of access to food.

The Universal Declaration of Human Rights, article 25, mentions both health and access to food as rights:

*"Everyone has the right to a standard of living adequate for the **health** and well-being of himself and of his family, **including food**, clothing, housing and medical care and necessary social services, and the right to security in the event of unemployment, sickness, disability, widowhood, old age or other lack of livelihood in circumstances beyond his control."*

The International Covenant on Economic, Social and Cultural Rights, meanwhile, provides the most comprehensive article on the right to health in international human rights law. Nutrition is mentioned as one of the determinants of health:

Article 12 of the Covenant recognizes the right of everyone to "the enjoyment of the highest attainable standard of physical and mental health." "Health" is understood not just as a right to be healthy, but as a right to control one's own health and body (including reproduction), and be free from interference such as torture or medical experimentation. States must protect this right by ensuring that everyone within their jurisdiction has access to the underlying determinants of health, such as clean water, sanitation, food, *nutrition* and housing, and through a comprehensive system of healthcare, which is available to everyone without discrimination, and economically accessible to all.

The UN Committee on Economic, Social, and Cultural Rights defines the "right to food" as follows:

*"The right to adequate food is realized when every man, woman and child, alone or in community with others, has physical and economic access at all times to adequate food or means for its procurement. **The right to adequate food shall therefore not be interpreted in a narrow or restrictive sense, which equates it with a minimum package of calories, proteins and other specific nutrients.** The right to adequate food will have to be realized progressively. However, States have a core obligation to take the necessary action to mitigate and alleviate hunger as provided for in paragraph 2 of article 11, even in times of natural or other disasters."*

However, as argued above, the prevention of chronic undernutrition, or stunting, should be a human right because of its widespread and irreversible lifelong consequences.

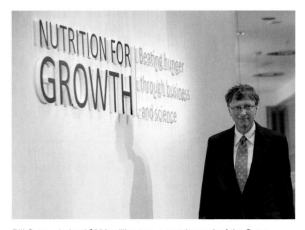

Bill Gates pledged $800 million to support the work of the Gates Foundation on nutrition and agriculture at the Nutrition for Growth conference
Source: The Children's Investment Fund Foundation

19

All stakeholders need to work together to prevent stunting

As thoroughly recognized by the Scaling Up Nutrition movement, all stakeholders need to work together to prevent stunting, including governments, the United Nations network, donor networks, civil society, and the private sector. These stakeholders must work together at national, regional and global level, in order to ensure access to adequate nutrition for all – in particular women and young children – and to prevent disease, which for example requires action by the healthcare sector as well as implementation of hygiene and sanitation measures. The call for all stakeholders to work together is easily made, but requires the laying out of a strong, localized roadmap that clearly identifies areas and responsibilities for action for the different stakeholder groups. Division of tasks within stakeholder groups should be done transparently. Tracking of implementation and progress is key to ensuring that the country stays on track relative to its roadmap.

It is increasingly recognized that the private sector, particularly the food industry, plays a critical role in achieving adequate nutrition and preventing stunting, and has to take that role even more seriously. The increase of

the average height of populations in the US, Europe, and parts of East Asia and Latin America in the second half of the 20th century coincided with dramatic economic development, and because access to healthcare, water and sanitation, and primary education was already good and did not change much during this period in these parts of the world, the improvement of nutritional status was to a large extent due to better access on the part of the lower economic strata of these populations to a more diverse diet, including improved, processed, complementary foods as well as animal-source foods such as dairy products. A good example is the average height of the Dutch male population, which increased from 165 cm in 1935 to 185 cm at the end of the 20th century. Increased height, which reflects better nutrition, is associated with higher IQ, a lower risk of cardiovascular diseases, but a slight increase of some kind of cancers, however, overall with a more healthy population.

The increase since the 1960s of cardiovascular diseases, obesity, type 2 diabetes, cancers, and other chronic diseases related to overconsumption of foods with a high content of fats and/or sugars but at the same time a low content of

The ten countries with the fastest annual reduction of stunting between 1990 and 2010

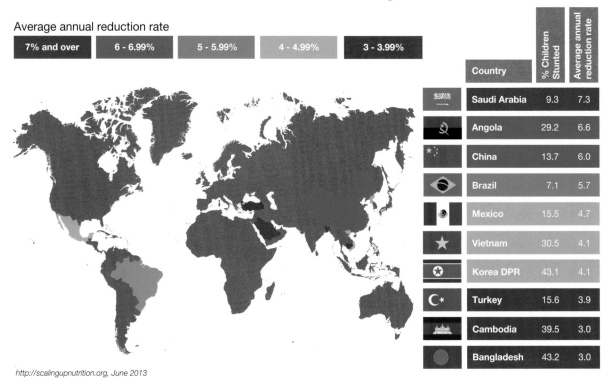

Average annual reduction rate

| 7% and over | 6 - 6.99% | 5 - 5.99% | 4 - 4.99% | 3 - 3.99% |

Country	% Children Stunted	Average annual reduction rate
Saudi Arabia	9.3	7.3
Angola	29.2	6.6
China	13.7	6.0
Brazil	7.1	5.7
Mexico	15.5	4.7
Vietnam	30.5	4.1
Korea DPR	43.1	4.1
Turkey	15.6	3.9
Cambodia	39.5	3.0
Bangladesh	43.2	3.0

http://scalingupnutrition.org, June 2013

vitamins, minerals and other essential nutrients, however, has further complicated the nutrition field. This requires corrective action from the food and beverage manufacturers.

This is also where the collaboration of the private sector with governments (who have legislative and norm-setting responsibilities) and civil society, donors and UN (who, for example, are important partners in healthcare, education and promoting consumer awareness of health and nutrition) is important, and the only way to ensure adequate nutrition for all.

Conclusion

There is an urgent need to give every child equal opportunities at the age of two. To achieve this, the prevention of stunting should be recognized as a human right. All stakeholders, including the private sector, need to collaborate to prevent stunting.

Because when...

Girls and women are well-nourished and have healthy newborn babies

Children receive proper nutrition and develop strong bodies and minds

Communities and nations are productive and stable

The world is a safer, more resilient and stronger place

Adolescents learn better and achieve higher grades in school

Families and communities emerge out of poverty

Young adults are better able to obtain work and earn more

http://scalingupnutrition.org, June 2013

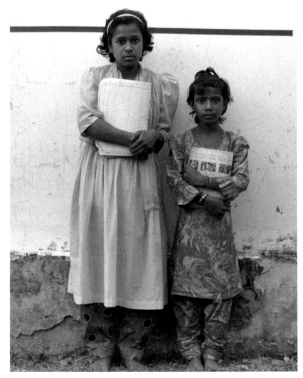

Two girls, Juhora Akter (left) and Asma Akter, who are both 12 years old, stand in front of a wall with a black tape line indicating the normal projected height for a 12-year-old child, in a rural area near the town of Shahrasti, Chandpur, Bangladesh
Source: UNICEF/NYHQ1997-0518/Gilles Vauclair

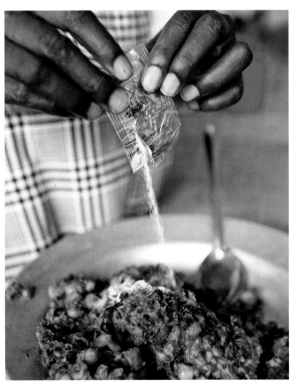

MixMe™ micronutrient powder being added to a meal to improve its nutritional value
Source: Mike Bloem Photography

21 A brief history of Human Rights

The General Assembly proclaims this Universal Declaration of Human Rights as a common standard of achievement for all peoples and all nations, to the end that every individual and every organ of society, keeping this Declaration constantly in mind, shall strive by teaching and education to promote respect for these rights and freedoms and by progressive measures, national and international, to secure their universal and effective recognition and observance, both among the peoples of Member States themselves and among the peoples of territories under their jurisdiction.

Declaration of Human Rights, 10 December 1948

The first known instance of a human rights agenda can be traced back to 539 BCE, when Cyrus the Great of Persia conquered the city of Babylon. In the wake of his triumph, he did something totally unexpected, freeing all the slaves in the city to return home. Moreover, he declared that the people under his rule should choose their own religion. The Cyrus Cylinder, a clay tablet containing these pronouncements, is one of the first human rights declarations in history.[1]

The idea of human rights spread quickly in the ancient world to India and Greece, and eventually Rome. The most important advances since then have included the 1215 British Magna Carta, which not only gave people new rights but also made the king subject to the law; the British 1628 Petition of Right, which formalized the rights of the people; the 1776 United States Declaration of Independence, which proclaimed the right to life, liberty and the pursuit of happiness; and the 1789 French Declaration of the Rights of Man and of the Citizen, a document stating that all citizens are equal under the law.[2]

In response to the crimes against humanity that were committed during the Second World War, the human rights revolution grew rapidly, subsuming claims from minorities, women, the politically oppressed, and marginal communities from around the globe.[3]

The human rights revolution began with a disarmingly simple idea: that every individual, whatever his or her nationality, political beliefs, or ethnic and religious heritage, possesses an inviolable right to be treated with dignity. From this basic claim grew many more, and ever since, the cascading effect of these initial rights claims has dramatically shaped world history.[4]

The Universal Declaration of Human Rights, the first document to list the 30 rights to which everyone is entitled, was adopted by the UN General Assembly on 10 December, 1948.[5]

The first draft of the Declaration was proposed in September 1948 with over 50 Member States participating in the final drafting. By its Resolution 217 A (III) of 10 December 1948, the General Assembly, meeting in Paris, adopted the Universal Declaration of Human Rights with eight nations abstaining from the vote but none dissenting. Hernán Santa Cruz of Chile, member of the drafting sub-Committee, wrote:

"I perceived clearly that I was participating in a truly significant historic event in which a consensus had been reached as to the supreme value of the human person, a value that did not originate in the decision of a worldly power, but rather in the fact of existing – which gave rise to the inalienable right to live free from want and oppression and to fully develop one's personality. In the Great Hall...there was an atmosphere of genuine solidarity and brotherhood among men and women from all latitudes, the like of which I have not seen again in any international setting."

The entire text of the Universal Declaration of Human Rights was composed in less than two years. At a time when the world was divided into Eastern and Western blocs, finding a common ground as to what should constitute the essence of the document proved a colossal task.[6]

1. Adapted from A Look at the Background of Human Rights, http://www.youthforhumanrights.org/what-are-human-rights/background-of-human-rights.html, July 2013

2. Adapted from A Look at the Background of Human Rights, http://www.youthforhumanrights.org/what-are-human-rights/background-of-human-rights.html, July 2013

3. Adapted from The Human Rights Revolution: Description http://global.oup.com/academic/product/the-human-rights-revolution-9780195333145?cc=gb&lang=en&tab=description, July 2013

4. Adapted from The Human Rights Revolution: Description http://global.oup.com/academic/product/the-human-rights-revolution-9780195333145?cc=gb&lang=en&tab=description, July 2013

5. Adapted from History of the Document http://www.un.org/en/documents/udhr/history.shtml, July 2013

6. Adapted from History of the Document http://www.un.org/en/documents/udhr/history.shtml, July 2013

Case study

Household Rice Expenditure and Maternal and Child Nutritional Status in Bangladesh

Increases in global food prices have raised concerns that the prevalence of malnutrition may increase, especially in developing countries. Rising food prices may decrease the ability of households to purchase food. Because poor households use a relatively large proportion of income to purchase food, increases in the price of food can directly affect the amount and type of food their income can buy, which can be reflected by decreased amounts of fat and vegetables in meals, elimination of some meals, and an overall reduction in dietary diversity. Because dietary diversity and animal-source foods are recognized as key components of high-quality diets, rising food prices can lead to a reduction in the quality of the diet. Reduced quality of the diet may adversely affect both nutrition and health over time. Previous studies have shown that increases in food prices lead to greater levels of stunting among children, decreased maternal micronutrient status, and impaired growth of infants.

In Bangladesh, poor rural families often deal with high food costs by purchasing primarily rice. The objective of [the current] study was to characterize the relationship between household expenditure on rice and non-rice foods with maternal and child malnutrition.

A recent study of data collected in the Nutritional Surveillance Project (NSP) in Bangladesh between 1992 and 2000 evaluated how changes in rice price affected child underweight. The percentage of underweight children declined in the situation where rice expenditures fell and households were able to spend more on non-rice foods. We sought to expand these investigations to evaluate the relationship between rice expenditure, non-rice expenditure, and household food expenditure and child stunting and maternal underweight between 2000 and 2005.

The results of [our] study show that households with higher expenditure on rice have increased odds of child stunting. Conversely, households with a higher expenditure on non-rice foods have decreased odds of child stunting. A similar relationship was observed between rice and non-rice food expenditures and maternal underweight. Previous studies have shown that changes in weekly expenditure on rice reflect changes in rice prices ... Previous studies have shown that the percentage of child underweight increases as rice expenditures rise. The present study extends these findings and suggests that higher expenditure on rice (reflecting higher food prices) increases the likelihood of developing child stunting.

Households with highest expenditures on rice and lower expenditures on non-rice foods have greater child malnutrition across all age categories up to 59 mo and greater maternal underweight. In a situation of global food prices, these findings suggest that there will be considerable impact upon the prevalence of child malnutrition and maternal underweight in developing countries.

Source: First published November 25, 2009, doi: 10.3945/jn.109.110718 J. Nutr. January 2010 vol. 140 no. 1 189S-194S [adapted and abridged]

Further reading

2013 Lancet Series on Maternal and Child Nutrition

Scaling Up Nutrition website: scalingupnutrition.org.

Copenhagen Consensus 2008/2012.

Baldi G, Martini E, Catharina M et al. Cost of the Diet (CoD) tool: First results from Indonesia and applications for policy discussion on food and nutrition security. Food Nutr Bull 2013;34:35S–42S.

de Pee S. Food Security. In: Caballero B. (ed.) Encyclopedia of Human Nutrition (3rd ed), vol. 2, pp. 353-360. Waltham, MA: Academic Press, 2013.

23 Case study

Malnutrition is treatable: access to nutrition services saves the life of a child (Uganda)

When 7-month-old Frank arrived at the Rubaga Hospital in Uganda in 2010, he was severely malnourished. He weighed only 7.5 pounds. Frank's aunt had less than $1 per week to feed and clothe him and his four other siblings. One of NuLife's 1,200 volunteers referred Frank to the hospital. (There are 54 NuLife-supported health facilities. NuLife is managed by University Research Co., LLC (URC) in partnership with the Uganda Ministry of Health (MOH). They are tasked with engaging multiple stakeholders to ensure nutrition care for people living with HIV/AIDS, pregnant and lactating women, and orphans and vulnerable children.

Frank was diagnosed with severe acute malnutrition. Staff prescribed and provided Frank with ready-to-use therapeutic food (RUTF) to treat his condition and enrolled him in an outpatient therapeutic care program.

His aunt also received nutrition counseling.

Frank's recovery was remarkable. After two months of RUTF he had exceeded his target weight by 20%. "Everybody gave Frank just two days to live when I first brought him, but now everybody wants to hold him and play with him," his aunt said. Frank would need to be taken back to hospital for regular follow-ups and more RUTF to ensure continued recovery.

Frank is just one of 16,000 individuals that have received treatment via NuLife. Project-supported healthcare facilities now assess close to 85% of HIV-positive individuals for malnutrition at admission, and sustainable processes are now in place allowing facilities to continue to address malnutrition. These NuLife achievements allow Ugandan health facilities to continue to treat children like Frank even after the project's completion in August 2011.

Source: Thousand Days Partnership, USA
http://www.thousanddays.org/success-story/malnutrition-is-treatable-access-to-nutrition-services-saves-the-life-of-a-ugandan-child/ Dec 2011 (abridged)

My personal view

Martin Bloem
Senior Nutritionist and WFP's Global Coordinator UNAIDS – United Nations World Food Program; Adjunct Associate Professor, – Johns Hopkins Bloomberg School of Public Health, Baltimore, USA; Adjunct Associate Professor, – Friedman School of Nutrition Science and Policy, Tufts University, Boston, USA

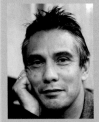

While the prevention of chronic undernutrition, or stunting, should be everyone's concern, because of the widespread consequences for schooling, economic development, long-term health etc, its prevention should ultimately result from better meeting children's nutrient requirements, and preventing an increase thereof, during the critical window of opportunity (conception to two years of age). Therefore, nutrition-specific actions, complemented with nutrition-sensitive approaches, are key. In the human rights documents, nutrition is only considered as a determinant to health, and the right to food only mentins access to "nutritious food" but none of the "human rights" documents recognizes the importance of nutrients in the sense that all required nutrients should be provided in adequate amounts. The particular need of children 6-24 months for nutrient-dense foods is very specific and the fact that these needs are difficult to meet from local foods for large segments of the world population urges for a discussion on the right to nutrients to prevent chronic undernutrition. Furthermore, meeting nutrient requirements of adolescent girls and women, particularly during pregnancy and lactation, should be prioritized as well, in order to protect their health and give their children the right start in life.

Food Security and Nutrition: Linkages and Complementarities

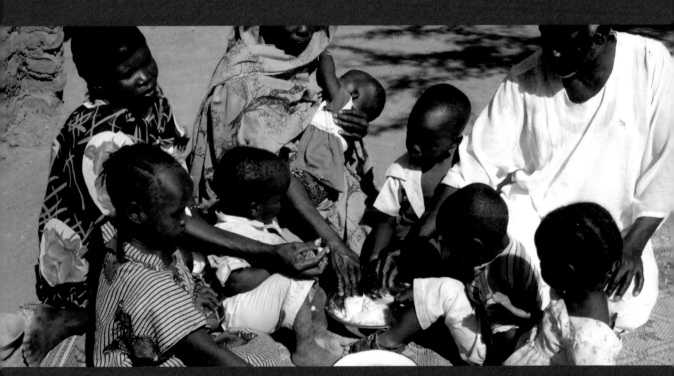

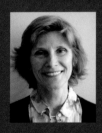

Marie Ruel

Division Director of Food Consumption and
Nutrition Division, International Food Policy
Research Institute (IFPRI) Washington DC, USA

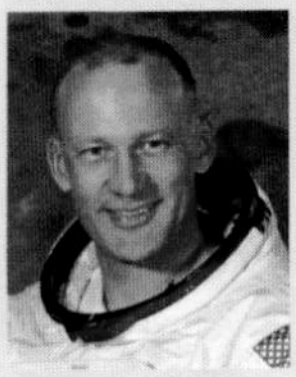

"If we can conquer space, we can conquer childhood hunger."

Buzz Aldrin

Key messages

- Food security and nutrition security are related but distinct concepts.

- Food security refers to having enough of the right foods at all times, and depends on the availability of food globally and locally, and on the household's and individual's access and proper utilization.

- Good nutrition (or nutrition security) also requires having enough of the right foods, but in addition, it requires having access to adequate feeding, caregiving and hygiene practices, as well as access to health, water and sanitation services. Nutrition security thus depends on having access to a healthy diet which provides all nutrients required for a healthy life, and being healthy so that the body can make optimal use of these nutrients for its different functions.

- Food security is necessary, but not sufficient, to ensure nutrition and to prevent childhood malnutrition. Children also need their caregivers to provide them with appropriate feeding, caregiving, hygiene, and health-seeking practices in order to grow, develop and stay healthy.

- Infants, young children, pregnant and breastfeeding women are especially vulnerable to malnutrition; nutrition interventions must focus on the critical 'First 1,000 Days' window of opportunity.

- Achieving food and nutrition security is a multi-faceted challenge which requires a multi-sectoral approach; food systems can play a critical role in protecting both food security and nutrition if careful attention is paid to targeting the poor, reducing inequalities, - including gender inequalities -, and incorporating nutrition goals and action where relevant.

Food and nutrition security: concepts and definitions

In the past half-century, the world has become increasingly aware of the challenges and threats to food security. This heightened awareness has been prompted by a range of well publicized humanitarian disasters and food price crises on the one hand and the burgeoning growth of the world's population and the changes in its dietary patterns on the other. Development organizations are increasingly concerned about food security and have focused their efforts on helping those who are not able to feed themselves sufficiently and adequately. Over the course of decades, these bodies have received the support of governments, private foundations and United Nations organizations. Many of their efforts have focused on provisioning food in situations of crisis or emergency, and increasingly on providing cash or food for development. Securing an adequate supply of food, however, is by no means the same thing as securing adequate nutrition. Investments in agricultural productivity and yields, for example, are not guaranteed to improve nutrition or health if they do not improve the poor's access both to enough calories and to

high-quality diets rich in essential nutrients. Even improving access to more and better food may be insufficient to prevent or reduce the persistently high rates of malnutrition found in the developing world if children are suffering from repeated episodes of diarrhea or other infections.

The distinction between food security and nutrition security is critically important because it affects what can be expected from the large, and in some cases growing, investments in boosting agriculture productivity and promoting global food security worldwide. For example, investments to stimulate agriculture production, especially those focused on staple cereals, although necessary, may not automatically result in better nutrition if they are not accompanied by complementary investments to improve access to health services for the poor.

Food security has been defined by the Food and Agriculture Organization of the United Nations (FAO) as existing "when all people, at all times, [have] physical, social and economic access to sufficient, safe and nutritious food to

The causes of malnutrition are interconnected

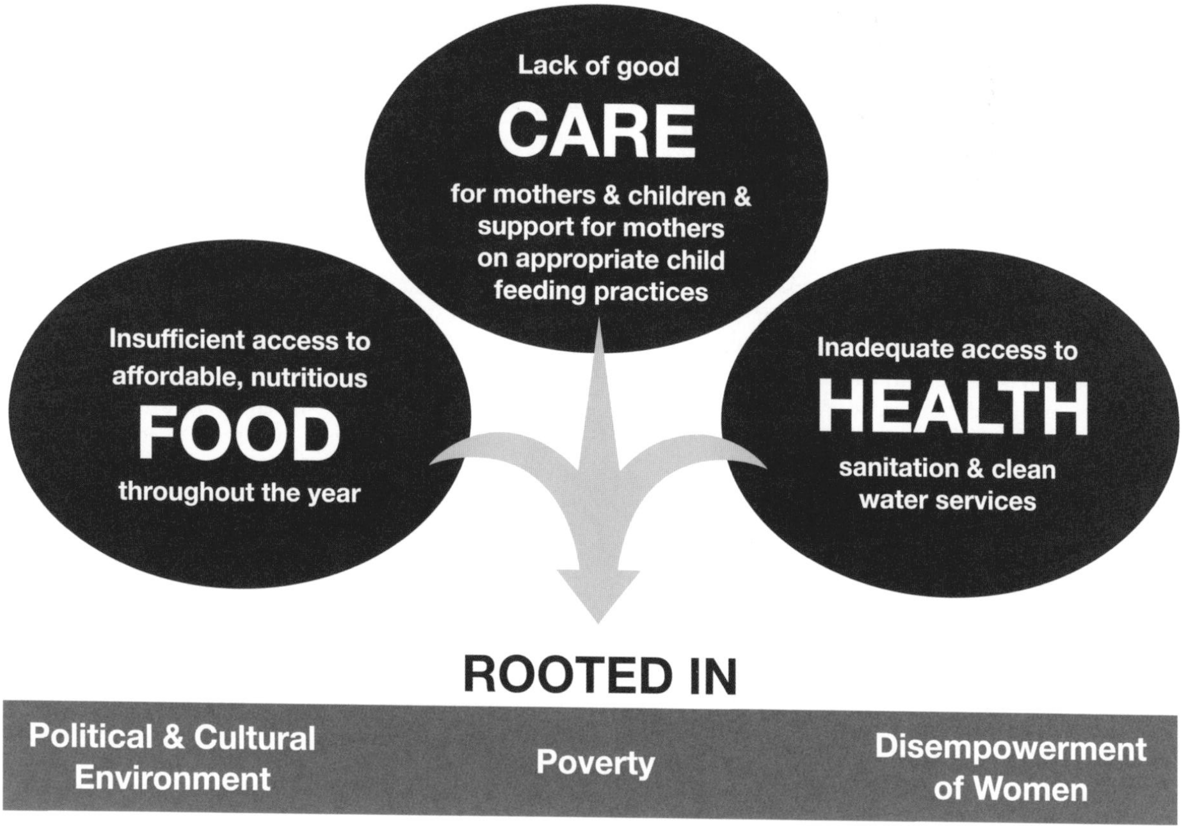

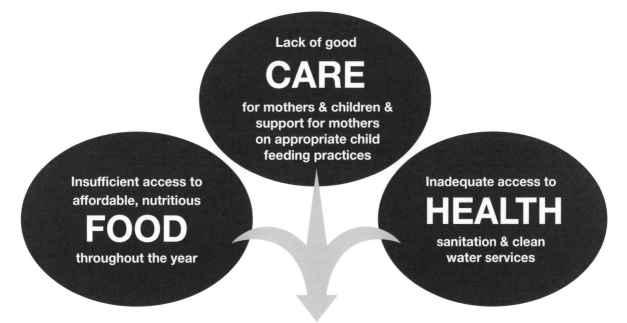

meet their dietary needs and food preferences for an active and healthy life" (FAO 1996, par. 1). Importantly, this definition stipulates that food should be available in sufficient *quantity* as well as in sufficient *quality*, should be *culturally acceptable*, and should be available *at all times* throughout the year.

Nutrition security, by contrast, exists when, in addition to having access to a healthy and balanced diet, people also have access to adequate caregiving practices and to a safe and clean environment that allows them to stay healthy and utilize the foods they eat effectively. For young children, for example, this means that they have enough of the right foods, and this includes breast milk for up to two years of age, along with appropriate quantity and quality of complementary foods starting at six months of age because breast milk can no longer fulfill all of the infant's nutrient needs after that age. In addition, young children also need caregivers who have the time, education, knowledge, physical and mental health, and nutritional well-being to care for them adequately. Adequate caregiving means that caregivers are able to attend to all their children's multiple needs, including adequate feeding, hygiene, health-seeking practices and supportive parenting. Finally, to be nutrition secure, young children must also be free of repeated (chronic) or acute infections, which interfere with absorption and utilization of food and nutrients for body functions.

Thus borrowing from both definitions, "food and nutrition security"can be defined as a situation that exists when all people at all times have physical, social and economic access to food, which is consumed in sufficient quantity and quality to meet their dietary needs, requirements for growth and food preferences, and is supported by an environment of adequate sanitation, health services and caregiving (United Nations Food and Agriculture Committee on World Food Security). This allows for appropriate utilization of food and nutrients by the body and therefore creates the conditions for a healthy and active life. Nutrition security therefore implies an optimal nutritional status.

To put this in more concrete terms, a person who has access to even the healthiest diet would not be able to benefit fully from that diet if he or she were ill or were living in the unsanitary conditions that foster illness. Poverty is often associated with insufficient food or foods of poor quality, in addition to suboptimal (or lack of) water and sanitation facilities, and compounded by an absence of knowledge of how to prevent contamination in the handling and preparation of food – which further compromises adequate nutrition, even if diets are adequate. People living in such circumstances are therefore drawn into a vicious cycle of infection which manifests itself

Linkages between food and nutrition security

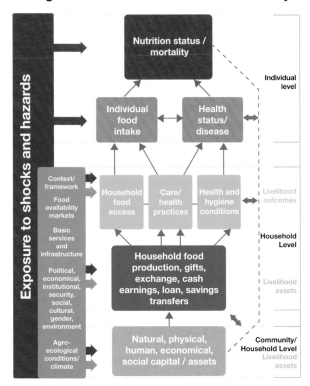

WFP Food and Nutrition Security Conceptual Framework (based on UNICEF conceptual framework for causes of malnutrition and DfID sustainable livelihoods framework). Reprinted with permission from WFP (2009) Comprehensive Food and Security Vulnerability Analysis Guidelines, Rome, Italy: WFP Available from www.wfp.org

by repeated bouts of illnesses, leading to poor nutrition, which in turn exacerbates poor health and susceptibility to infections, and perpetuates poverty.

Many global, national and local factors compromise the choices that poor populations have regarding their food consumption and diets. These include global changes in the food systems such as food and oil price volatility, climate change and resulting water shortages, and natural disasters affecting agriculture productivity, as well as conflicts and emergencies. At the local level, bad harvests, poor agricultural and husbandry practices, inappropriate procedures for the packaging and storage of food, and inadequate distribution mechanisms affect poor farmers' food production and income, as well as their purchasing power. Food and nutrition insecurity are the result of inequity.

Most vulnerable of all are infants and young children during their first two years of life, and women when they are pregnant or breastfeeding. The vulnerability of these two groups comes from the fact that they have very high requirements for essential nutrients (e.g. vitamin A, iron, zinc, iodine, etc.) during these periods. For children, these nutrients are necessary for them to grow and for their brain to develop; for pregnant women, they are necessary because they have to provide extra calories and nutrients to their growing fetus; and for lactating mothers, they are necessary because the mothers are producing breast milk, and this requires consuming extra calories and micronutrients so that they can produce enough milk and for the milk to be of adequate quality.

The critical importance of this period (pregnancy, lactation and first two years of a child's life), which is now referred to as the "First 1,000 Days" from conception to the two years of age, was made clear in a groundbreaking piece of research published by The Lancet Journal in 2008 and further emphasized in a new Series on Maternal and Child Nutrition published in the same journal in 2013. Both series highlight that not only is this 1,000-day period the time when mothers and children are most at risk of malnutrition, but that it is also the period when they can most benefit from interventions to prevent the negative consequences of malnutrition. In fact, what happens during the first 1,000 days determines the future of an individual, and nutritional damage that happens during this period is largely irreversible. Children undernourished during this period are shown to have delays in mental development, are less likely to perform well and to stay in school, have less skilled jobs and lower income in adulthood, and are at increased risk of developing problems of overweight and obesity and other chronic diseases such as heart diseases, diabetes and some types of cancers in adulthood.

"Food security exists when all people, at all times, have physical and economic access to sufficient safe and nutritious food that meets their dietary needs and food preferences for an active and healthy life."

-1996 World Food Summit

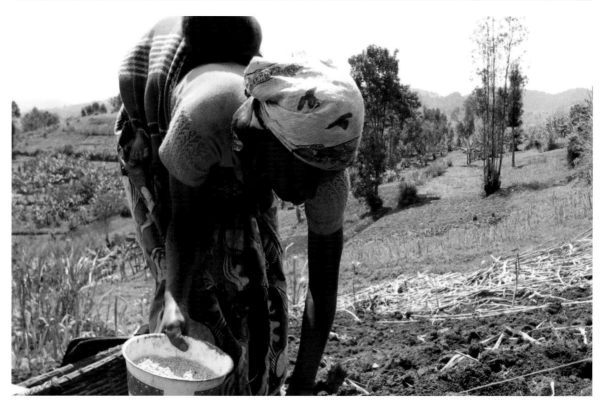

Mother working in agriculture (with child)
Source: One Acre Fund

The four dimensions of food security

The definition of food security highlights the fact that food security is a multi-faceted problem, which includes four key dimensions: availability, access, utilization and stability. The four dimensions of food security are defined as:

Physical AVAILABILITY of food	Food availability addresses the "supply side" of food security and is determined by the level of food production, stock levels and net trade.
Economic and physical ACCESS to food	An adequate supply of food at the national or international level does not in itself guarantee household level food security. Concerns about insufficient food access have resulted in a greater policy focus on incomes, expenditure, markets and prices in achieving food security objectives.
Food UTILIZATION	Utilization is commonly understood as the way the body makes the most of various nutrients in the food. Sufficient energy and nutrient intake by individuals is the result of good care and feeding practices, food preparation, diversity of the diet and intra-household distribution of food. Combined with good biological utilization of food consumed, this determines the nutritional status of individuals.
STABILITY of the other three dimensions over time	Even if your food intake is adequate today, you are still considered to be food insecure if you have inadequate access to food on a periodic basis, risking a deterioration of your nutritional status. Adverse weather conditions, political instability, or economic factors (unemployment, rising food prices) may have an impact on your food security status.

Source: United Nations Food and Agriculture Organization (FAO)

For food security objectives to be realized, all four dimensions must be fulfilled simultaneously.

The four dimensions of food security and their determinants

Availability	Access	Utilization	Stability
• **Domestic production** • **Import capacity** • **Food stocks** • **Food aid**	• **Income, purchasing power, own production** • **Transport and market infrastructure** • **Food distribution**	• **Food safety and qualtiy** • **Clean water** • **Health and sanitation** • **Care, feeding and health-seeking practices**	• **Weather variability, seasonality** • **Price fluctuations** • **Political factors** • **Economic factors**

Source: Adapted from FAO

Food security analysts have also defined two general types of food insecurity: *chronic* and *transitory* food insecurity. These are defined on the basis of their temporality, severity and rate of recurrence.

	CHRONIC FOOD INSECURITY	TRANSITORY FOOD INSECURITY
Is...	long-term or persistent.	short-term and temporary.
Occurs when...	people are unable to meet their minimum food requirements over a sustained period of time.	there is a sudden drop in the ability to produce or access enough food to maintain a good nutritional status.
Results from...	extended periods of poverty, lack of assets and inadequate access to productive or financial resources.	short-term shocks and fluctuations in food availability and access, including year-to-year variations in domestic food production, food prices and household incomes.
Can be overcome with...	typical long-term development measures also used to address poverty, such as education or access to productive resources, such as credit. People may also need more direct access to food to enable them to raise their productive capacity.	transitory food insecurity is relatively unpredictable and can emerge suddenly. This makes planning and programming more difficult and requires different capacities and types of intervention, including early warning capacity and safety net programs (see Box 1).

Seasonal food insecurity is yet another term. This is used to refer to food insecurity of limited duration linked to cyclical patterns of inadequate availability and access to food. Seasonal food insecurity is usually associated with seasonal fluctuations in climate, cropping patterns, work opportunities (labor demand), income, and patterns of diseases.

Chapter Two

The causes and consequences of food insecurity

Food insecurity is not a new phenomenon. The effects of natural and man-made disasters have always placed a severe burden on food systems, and there have been few societies that have existed without the fear of famine, or the memory of it.

Famine is also a highly topical subject – as witnessed in the 2011 drought in the Horn of Africa. Figures compiled by the UK Department for International Development (DfID) suggest that between 50,000 and 100,000 people, more than half of them children under five, died as a result of the drought. A total of 13 million are believed to have been affected by the disaster, with livelihoods, livestock and local market systems all caught up in a complex chain of interdependency and suffering. According to a report published by Save the Children and Oxfam, and entitled *A Dangerous Delay*, many of the deaths could have been prevented had governments and humanitarian agencies been quicker to read the warning signs. "Waiting for a situation to reach crisis point before responding is the wrong way to address chronic vulnerability and recurrent drought in places like the Horn of Africa," the report concluded. "The international community must change the way it operates to meet the challenge of recurrent crises … Long-term development work is best placed to respond to drought."

Even in situations in which natural and man-made disasters are not placing intolerable strain on food systems, however, challenges to food security remain in many parts of the world. Lack of water for irrigation, poor soil, inadequate agricultural practices and lack of appropriate tools and seeds can make it difficult to improve yields and efficiency in the production of nutritious foods. Lack of land itself is another major factor, as is, of course, lack of capital. Unsuitable transport systems and inappropriate storage practices can further compromise food stocks whose nutritional value and quality may already be questionable.

In addition to these factors, which affect the availability of food globally, there are cultural practices and beliefs that determine how food is allocated to different individuals within the household – for example the practice of men eating before women and children in some parts of the world (and consuming the choicest and most nutritious elements in a meal because they are the family breadwinner and perceived to need more food, and more of the high-quality foods, than other family members); or the cultural beliefs that some foods (such as eggs in Ghana) should not be given to young children because this may make them thieves when they grow up; or mangoes, which could be an excellent source of vitamin A for young children, but are not given to them in some cultures because these fruits are thought to cause diarrhea.

Another critical factor that determines whether households are food secure or not is women – their social status, their access to resources, and their ability to make key decisions regarding allocation of income and other resources, such as food, within the household. It has been shown over and over again that men and women use resources differently, and that when women have more resources under their control (e.g. income), they are more likely than men to protect the food security of their family and to invest in the health, education and nutrition of their children. For decades now, women have been referred to as being "the key to food security"; they are also critically important for protecting the health and nutrition of their children. Women's education, their physical and mental health, and nutritional well-being, as well as the time they have available, are all essential ingredients for ensuring their family's food security. These factors are equally important determinants of how women can take care of their young children's needs, protect them from infectious diseases, and help them grow and develop into healthy adults, which in turn will equip them to more successfully achieve food security for their own family in the future.

It would be incorrect, however, to assume that food insecurity problems are limited exclusively to the developing

Food insecurity, malnutrition and poverty are deeply interrelated phenomena

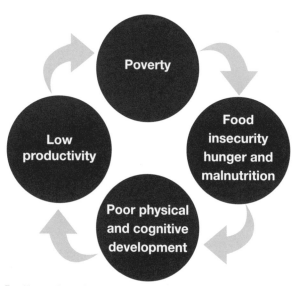

Food insecurity, malnutrition and poverty are deeply interrelated phonemena

world. Food insecurity and deficiencies of essential nutrients such as iron are widespread among the poorest segments of the population in many affluent countries. As described in the chapter on obesity in this book, in developed countries, food insecurity often leads resource-constrained households to feed their families cheap, calorie-dense fast foods instead of fresh fruits and vegetables, meat and dairy, which are typically much more expensive. As a result, food insecure households in the developed world often have poor quality diets containing high levels of saturated fat, refined sugar and salt, which lead to severe problems of overweight and obesity not only in adults but also in children. Obesity and overweight lead to stigma and social problems, and more importantly, they are the most significant risk factors for a series of health problems including cardiovascular diseases, diabetes and some forms of cancer. Food insecurity and malnutrition are not just problems of poor countries; governments throughout the world need to find appropriate solutions to protect the food security and nutrition of their population.

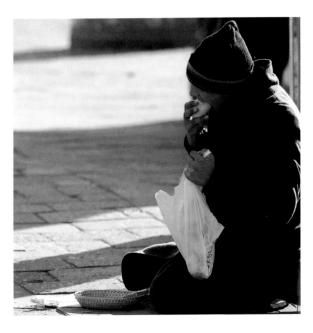

How households cope with food insecurity, and the consequences for health and nutrition

Deterioration of household food security

Livelihood	Diversification / change in livelihood activities	Reduced expenditure on non-essential or luxury items. Beginning to sell non-productive / disposable assets	Children drop out of school. Emigration (from rural to urban areas)	Increased use of child labor. Begin to borrow / purchase on credit. Become indebted	Selling of productive assets	Selling of all assets	Reduce expenditures on essential items (e.g. food, water etc.)	Engage in illegal / health-threatening activities as last resort coping
Food-related	Change to cheaper, lower-quality and less-preferred foods	Reduced diversity of food. Poor nutrient intake. Favor certain HH members over others for consumption	Reduced size / number of meals	Consume wild foods / immature crops / seeds. Send HH members elsewhere to eat (e.g., neigbors)	Begging for food	Skip entire days without eating	Eat items not eaten in the past / not part of normal diet (e.g. plants, insects etc.)	

Consequences for health and nutrition

Health outcome	Depletion of body nutrient stores and lowered immunity	Appearance of clinical symptoms such as wasting, night blindness, anemia, increased morbidity and failure to grow	Increased early childhood mortality	Increased overall mortality

Changes in livelihood, food selection and consumption, and nutritional status and health outcome when households descend into stress and distress.
Reprinted with permission from Klotz C, de Pee S, Thorne-Lyman A, Kraemer K and Bloem MW. Nutrition in a perfect storm: Why micronutrient malnutrition will be a widespread health consequence of high food prices. Sight and Life Magazine(2008) 2: 6–13. Adapted from D. Maxwell, R. Caldwell. The Coping Strategies Index: Field Methods Manual, Nairobi: CARE Eastern and Central Africa Regional Management and World Food Programme, 2nd ed, Jan 2008.

Hunger[1] statistics

1) 870 million people in the world do not have enough to eat. This number has fallen by 130 million since 1990, but progress slowed after 2008.

(Source: State of Food Insecurity in the World, FAO, 2012)

2) The vast majority of hungry people (98 percent) live in developing countries, where almost 15% of the population is undernourished.

(Source: State of Food Insecurity in the World, FAO, 2012)

3) Asia and the Pacific have the largest share of the world's hungry people (some 563 million) but the trend is downward.

(Source: State of Food Insecurity in the World, FAO, 2012)

4) Women make up a little over half of the world's population, but they account for over 60 percent of the world's hungry.

(Source: Strengthening efforts to eradicate hunger..., ECOSOC, 2007)

5) 66 million primary-school-age children attend classes hungry across the developing world, with 23 million in Africa alone.

(Source: Two Minutes to Learn About School Meals, WFP, 2012)

[1] The term "hunger" is commonly used to refer to "food insecurity"

Malnutrition statistics

1) Undernutrition (including fetal growth restriction, stunting, wasting, and deficiencies of vitamin A and zinc along with sub-optimal breastfeeding) contributes to more than 3 million deaths of children per year – up to 45% of the global total.

(Source: Lancet Paper 1 (Black et al 2013)

2) Roughly 100 million children under 5 years of age are underweight (16%)

(Source: Lancet Paper 1 (Black et al 2013)

3) There are still 165 million children stunted in the world (26% or 1 in 4 children) and at least 52 million wasted (8%)

(Source: Lancet Paper 1 (Black et al 2013)

4) In 2011, 43 million children younger than 5 years, or 7%, were overweight – a 54% increase from an estimated 28 million in 1990.

(Source: Lancet Paper 1 (Black et al 2013)

> *Maternal and child undernutrition is the cause of more than 3 million deaths annually*
>
> **(Black et al,** Lancet Series 2013)

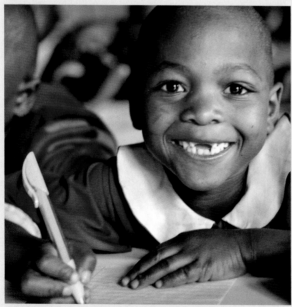

A girl happy to learn in a classroom in Kenya in 2009
Source: Mike Bloem Photography

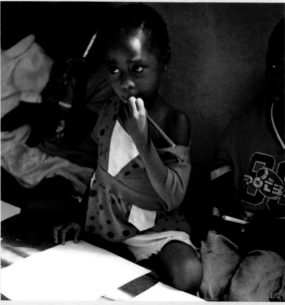

Girl learning in an orphanage classroom in Port-au-Prince, Haiti
Source: Mike Bloem Photography

33

UNICEF Conceptual Framework

The UNICEF framework, which the nutrition community has been using for programming for the past 25 years, identifies three levels of causes of undernutrition

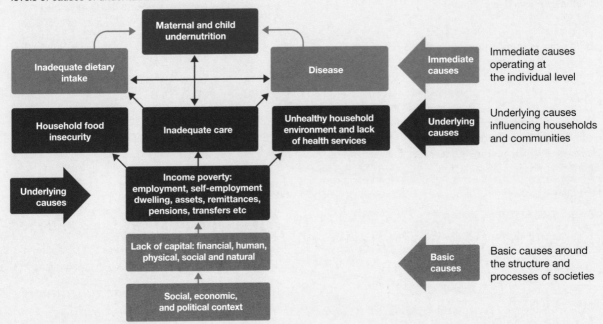

The UNICEF conceptual framework

More than two decades ago, UNICEF developed a conceptual framework that identifies the causes of undernutrition. The nutrition community has used it extensively ever since because it provides a useful visualization of the multiple factors that affect maternal and child undernutrition. The framework is particularly useful to illustrate the different levels of factors that affect nutrition – for example factors at the national, community, household and individual levels – and refers to basic, underlying and direct determinants of undernutrition. Some variations of the models also show examples of interventions that can be used to address some of the determinants of undernutrition at these different levels.

The UNICEF conceptual framework is as relevant today as it was then, but it is now influenced by recent shifts and exciting developments in the field of nutrition.

Strengthened by new evidence, an understanding of the short- and long-term consequences of undernutrition has evolved. There is even stronger confirmation that undernutrition can trap children, families, communities and nations in an intergenerational cycle of poor nutrition,

illness and poverty. More is known about the mechanisms that link inadequate growth due to nutritional deficiencies before the age of 2 with impaired brain development and subsequent reduced performance in school. And there is clearer, more comprehensive evidence of the need to promote optimal growth during this critical period to avoid an elevated risk of non-communicable diseases, such as cardiovascular disease, in adulthood and even in the next generation.

The UNICEF conceptual framework defines nutrition and captures the multifactorial causality of undernutrition (Figure 1). Nutritional status is influenced by three broad factors: food, health and care. Optimal nutritional status results when children have access to affordable, diverse, nutrient-rich food; appropriate maternal and child-care practices; adequate health services; and a healthy environment including safe water, sanitation and good hygiene practices. These factors directly influence nutrient intake and the presence of disease. The interaction between undernutrition and infection creates a potentially lethal cycle of worsening illness and deteriorating nutritional status.

Food, health and care are affected by social, economic and political factors. The combination and relative importance of these factors differ from country to country.

Understanding the immediate and underlying causes of undernutrition in a given context is critical to delivering appropriate, effective and sustainable solutions and adequately meeting the needs of the most vulnerable people.

Immediate causes of undernutrition

At the immediate level, the two main causes of undernutrition are a lack of appropriate food and nutrient intake, and disease. Undernutrition can result from consuming too few nutrients or from having repeated infections, which increase nutrient requirements and prevent the body from absorbing those consumed, or both.

The infection-undernutrition cycle

An estimated one third of deaths among children under age 5 are attributed to undernutrition. Undernutrition puts children at far greater risk of death and severe illness due to common childhood infections, such as pneumonia, diarrhea, malaria, HIV and AIDS and measles. A child who is severely underweight is 9.5 times more likely to die of diarrhea than a child who is not, and for a stunted child the risk of death is 4.6 times higher.

Undernutrition weakens the immune system, putting children at higher risk of more severe, frequent and prolonged bouts of illness. Undernutrition is also a consequence of repeated infections, which may further worsen the child's nutritional status at a time of greater nutritional needs. This interaction between undernutrition and infection creates a potentially lethal cycle of worsening illness and deteriorating nutritional status.

Critical nutrition interventions that break this cycle include promoting optimal breastfeeding practices, encouraging micronutrient supplementation and reducing the incidence of low birth weight. For example, infants not breastfed are 15 times more likely to die from pneumonia and 11 times more likely to die from diarrhea than children who are exclusively breastfed. Similarly, all-cause mortality is 14 times higher for infants not breastfeeding than for exclusively breastfed children.

Today's concerted focus on reducing stunting reflects an improved understanding of the importance of undernutrition during the most critical period of development in early life and of the long-term consequences extending into adulthood. Evidence from 54 low- and middle-income countries indicates that growth faltering on average begins during pregnancy and continues to about 24 months of age. This loss in linear growth is not recovered, and catch-up growth later on in childhood is minimal.

While the original UNICEF conceptual framework reflected a focus on children of preschool age, there is now more emphasis on policies and programs that support action before the age of 2 years, especially on maternal nutrition and health and appropriate infant and young child feeding and care practices.

Adequate maternal nutrition, health and physical status are crucial to prevent child undernutrition. Pregnancy increases nutrient needs, and protein, energy, vitamin and mineral deficiencies are common during pregnancy. Deficiencies are not solely the result of inadequate dietary intake: Disease can impair absorption of nutrients and reduce appetite, and environmental and psychosocial stress affecting the mother can contribute to child undernutrition. Poor maternal nutrition impairs fetal development and contributes to low birth weight, subsequent stunting and other forms of undernutrition.

Undernourished girls have a greater likelihood of becoming undernourished mothers who in turn have a greater chance of giving birth to low birth weight babies, perpetuating an intergenerational cycle. This cycle can be compounded further in young mothers, especially adolescent girls who begin childbearing before attaining adequate growth and development. Short intervals between pregnancies and having several children may accumulate or exacerbate nutrition deficits, passing these deficiencies on to the children.

Low birth weight is associated with increased morbidity and mortality: An estimated 60 to 80 percent of neonatal deaths occur among low birth weight babies (2005 estimate). In South Asia, an estimated 28 percent of infants are born with low birth weight.

(Source: Improving Child Nutrition, The achievable imperative for global progress. UNICEF 2013)

Food system interventions for better nutrition

Policy environment and development priorities

FOOD SYSTEM ELEMENTS	NUTRITION OPPORTUNITIES	POLICY TOOLS
Production "up to the farm gate" (R&D, inputs, production, farm management)	• Sustainable intensification of production • Nutrition-promoting farming systems, agronomic practices and crops - Micronutrient fertilizers - Biofortified crops - Integrated farming systems, including fisheries and forestry - Crop and livestock diversification • Stability for food security and nutrition - Grain reserves and storage - Crop and livestock insurance • Nutrition education - School and home gardens • Nutrient preserving on-farm storage	• Food and agricultural policies to promote availability, affordability, diversity and quality • Nutrition-oriented agricultural research on crops, livestock and production systems • Promotion of school and home gardens
Post-harvest supply chain "from the farm gate to retailer" (marketing, storage, trade, processing, retailing)	• Nutrient-preserving processing, packaging, transport and storage • Reduced waste and increased technical and economic efficiency • Food fortification • Reformulation for better nutrition (e.g. elimination of trans fats) • Food safety	• Regulation and taxation to promote efficiency, safety, quality, diversity • Research and promotion of innovation in product formulation, processing and transport
Consumers (advertizing, labelling, education, safety nets)	• Nutrition information and health claims • Product labelling • Consumer education • Social protection for food security and nutrition - General food assistance programs and subsidies - Targeted food assistance (prenatal, children, elderly, etc.)	• Food assistance programs • Food price incentives • Nutrition regulations • Nutrition education and information campaigns

Economic, social, cultural and physical environment

Gender roles and environmental sustainability

AVAILABLE, ACCESSIBLE, DIVERSE, NUTRITIOUS FOODS

Health, food safety, education, sanitation and infrastructure

Source: FAO

What can food systems do to enhance food security and nutrition?

Food systems produce, market, store, trade, process, retail, and promote food for consumers to acquire and use to feed their families. Food systems also provide livelihood and income to large amounts of the population around the globe, including many of the world's poorest. The latest Food and Agriculture Organization (FAO)'s State of Food and Agriculture report, published in 2013, argues that "food systems – from agricultural inputs and production, through processing, marketing and retailing, to consumption – can promote more nutritious and sustainable diets for everyone" (p. 3). The report also highlights that while the nature and causes of food insecurity and malnutrition are complex and diverse, a common denominator for both conditions is a nutritionally deficient diet. For this reason, the food system provides an opportunity to address both food insecurity and malnutrition, but in order to do so, the food system needs to be re-shaped to be more nutrition-sensitive. The diagram below presents the framework adopted by FAO, which highlights opportunities for incorporating nutrition considerations into different elements of the food system. More specific guidance has also been developed on how to improve nutrition through agriculture programs and policies.

"Of course, addressing malnutrition requires interventions not only in the food system, but also in the health, sanitation, education and other sectors. Integrated actions are needed across the health, education and agriculture sectors"

FAO, *2013, p. 3*

Key recommendations for Improving Nutrition through Agriculture

Food systems provide for all people's nutritional needs, while at the same time contributing to economic growth. The food and agriculture sector has the primary role in feeding people well by increasing availability, affordability, and consumption of diverse, safe, nutritious foods and diets, aligned with dietary recommendations and environmental sustainability. Applying these principles helps strengthen resilience and contributes to sustainable development.

Agricultural programs and investments can strengthen impact on nutrition if they:

1. Incorporate explicit nutrition objectives and indicators into their design, and track and mitigate potential harms, while seeking synergies with economic, social and environmental objectives.

2. Assess the context at the local level, to design appropriate activities to address the types and causes of malnutrition, including chronic or acute undernutrition, vitamin and mineral deficiencies, and obesity and chronic disease. Context assessment can include potential food resources, agro-ecology, seasonality of production and income, access to productive resources such as land, market opportunities and infrastructure, gender dynamics and roles, opportunities for collaboration with other sectors or programs, and local priorities.

3. Target the vulnerable and improve equity through participation, access to resources, and decent employment. Vulnerable groups include smallholders, women, youth, the landless, urban dwellers, the unemployed.

4. Collaborate and coordinate with other sectors (health, environment, social protection, labor, water and sanitation, education, energy) and programs, through joint strategies with common goals, to address concurrently the multiple underlying causes of malnutrition.

5. Maintain or improve the natural resource base (water, soil, air, climate, biodiversity), critical to the livelihoods and resilience of vulnerable farmers and to sustainable food and nutrition security for all. Manage water resources in particular to reduce vector-borne illness and to ensure sustainable, safe household water sources.

6. Empower women by ensuring access to productive resources, income opportunities, extension services and information, credit, labor and time-saving technologies (including energy and water services), and supporting their voice in household and farming decisions. Equitable opportunities to earn and learn should be compatible with safe pregnancy and young child feeding.

7. Facilitate production diversification, and increase production of nutrient-dense crops and small-scale livestock (for example, horticultural products, legumes, livestock and fish at a small scale, under-utilized crops, and biofortified crops). Diversified production systems are important to vulnerable producers to enable resilience to climate and price shocks, more diverse food consumption, reduction of seasonal food and income fluctuations, and greater and more gender-equitable income generation.

8. Improve processing, storage and preservation to retain nutritional value, shelf-life, and food safety, to reduce seasonality of food insecurity and post-harvest losses, and to make healthy foods convenient to prepare.

9. Expand markets and market access for vulnerable groups, particularly for marketing nutritious foods or products vulnerable groups have a comparative advantage in producing. This can include innovative promotion (such as marketing based on nutrient content), value addition, access to price information, and farmer associations.

10. Incorporate nutrition promotion and education around food and sustainable food systems that builds on existing local knowledge, attitudes and practices. Nutrition knowledge can enhance the impact of production and income in rural households, especially important for women and young children, and can increase demand for nutritious foods in the general population.

These recommendations have been formulated following an extensive review of available guidance on agriculture programming for nutrition, conducted by FAO (see: http://www.fao.org/docrep/017/aq194e/aq194e00.htm), and through consultation with a broad range of partners (CSOs, NGOs, government staff, donors, UN agencies) in particular through the Ag2Nut Community of Practice. They are also referred to as "guiding principles" by some partners.

Agriculture programs and investments need to be supported by an enabling policy environment if they are to contribute to improving nutrition. Governments can encourage improvements in nutrition through agriculture by taking into consideration the five policy actions below.

Food and agriculture policies can have a better impact on nutrition if they:

1. Increase incentives (and decrease disincentives) for availability, access, and consumption of diverse, nutritious and safe foods through environmentally sustainable production, trade, and distribution. The focus needs to be on horticulture, legumes, and small-scale livestock and fish – foods which are relatively unavailable and expensive, but nutrient-rich – and vastly under-utilized as sources of both food and income.

2. Monitor dietary consumption and access to safe, diverse, and nutritious foods. The data could include food prices of diverse foods, and dietary consumption indicators for vulnerable groups.

3. Include measures that protect and empower the poor and women. Safety nets that allow people to access nutritious food during shocks or seasonal times when income is low; land tenure rights; equitable access to productive resources; market access for vulnerable producers (including information and infrastructure). Recognizing that a majority of the poor are women, ensure equitable access to all of the above for women.

4. Develop capacity in human resources and institutions to improve nutrition through the food and agriculture sector, supported with adequate financing.

5. Support multi-sectoral strategies to improve nutrition within national, regional, and local government structures.

The present key recommendations for Improving Nutrition through Agriculture target policy-makers and program planners. These recommendations are based on the current global context, and may be updated over time as challenges and opportunities to improve nutrition present themselves.

My personal view

Marie Ruel
Division Director of Food Consumption and Nutrition Division, IFPRI. Washington DC, USA

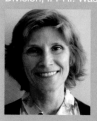

Food security and nutrition security are two complex, interrelated phenomena that result from a series of factors – some that are common to both conditions and others that are not.

In spite of the commonalities and close linkages between the two phenomena, however, in my view, it is unwise to combine the two concepts into one named "food and nutrition security". I would prefer to see food security and nutrition (or nutrition security) remain as two distinct, yet clearly related phenomena.

The first reason is that the combined concept of food and nutrition security (as defined in this chapter) is very broad and may be difficult to operationalize. It may be particularly difficult, for instance, to define policies and programs that would encompass all the factors that need to be addressed to support both food and nutrition security, let alone identifying the right set of indicators to properly measure the impact of these actions on relevant food security and nutrition outcomes.

Secondly, not all food security and agriculture-focused policies and programs necessarily need to be accountable for improving nutrition. In some cases, it may be more cost-effective to co-locate programs aimed at tackling poverty and food insecurity with programs specifically focused on improving nutrition and to target the same households and individuals for maximum impact.

Even more importantly, by combining nutrition with food security, we run the risk of seeing nutrition lose its momentum and become absorbed by (and lost within) the broader umbrella of food security. We need to move away from food security being perceived as synonymous to nutrition, and for this, we need to keep the concepts distinct from each other. We also need to correct the wrong perception that if more food could be produced and food security ensured, malnutrition would automatically disappear.

As highlighted in this chapter, more food and more of the right quality foods are necessary, but not enough, to improve nutrition: investments aimed at boosting agriculture production and productivity and at ensuring food security of all people need to be accompanied by renewed efforts to reduce the burden of infectious diseases and increase poor people's access to health, water, sanitation and education services. Most importantly, progress in nutrition will be made if we can tackle inequality in all its forms, starting with gender inequalities.

Further reading

Quisumbing AR, Brown LR, Sims Feldstein H et al. *Women: the key to food security. Food Policy Report.* Washington, DC: International Food Policy Research Institute, 1995. And: *Women, still the key to food security.* IFPRI Issue Brief 33, 2005.

Food and Agriculture Organization. *The state of food insecurity in the world 2012. Economic growth is necessary but not sufficient to accelerate reduction of hunger and malnutrition.* Rome: Food and Agriculture Organization, 2012.

Food and Agriculture Organization. *The state of food and agriculture 2013. Food systems for better nutrition.* Rome: Food and Agriculture Organization, 2013.

Pinstrup-Andersen P. *Food security: Definition and measurement.* Food Security 2009;1(1): 5–7.

Pinstrup-Andersen P. *The food system and its interaction with human health nutrition. Leveraging agriculture for improved nutrition and health.* 2020 Conference brief 13. Washington, DC: International Food Policy Research Institute, 2011.

Ruel M T, Alderman H and the Maternal and Child Nutrition Study Group. *Nutrition-sensitive interventions and programs: How can they help accelerate progress in improving maternal and child nutrition?* Published online, The Lancet, 6 June 2013.

Chapter Three

Hidden Hunger in the Developed World

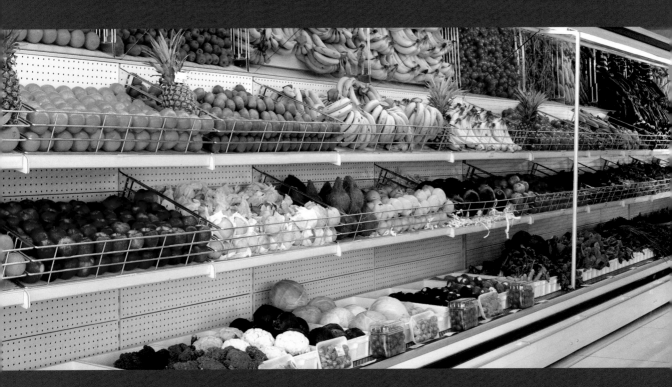

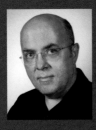

Hans Konrad Biesalski

Department of Biological Chemistry and Nutrition,

University of Hohenheim, Stuttgart, Germany

"The food you eat can be either the safest and most powerful form of medicine or the slowest form of poison."

Ann Wigmore, *Lithuanian holistic health practitioner, nutritionist and health educator.*

Key messages

Solutions are available: Many countries have implemented mandatory or voluntary fortification of folic acid, vitamin D or iodine. The experience of many countries indicates that the fortification of staple or processed foods may be an efficient way to provide an adequate intake of micronutrients.

The term "hidden hunger" has gained significant currency among nutrition scientists and policy-makers in recent years. In its broadest sense, it denotes a chronic lack of micronutrients – vitamins and minerals – whose effects may not be immediately apparent and whose consequences may be long-term and profound.

While much groundbreaking research into the subject of hidden hunger has been conducted in the last two decades, many questions remain regarding the extent and implications of this phenomenon and the best means of tackling it. From today's perspective, however, it is clear that hidden hunger is a growing threat to public health, both in the developing and the developed worlds.

The following chapter provides a short introduction and examples to this topic, which is complex, ramified, and the subject of considerable scientific attention and controversy as this book goes to press.

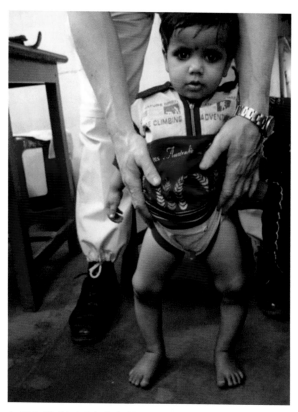

A child with rickets in India in 2006. This non-communicable disease is associated with vitamin D deficiency and results in irreversible malformation of the skeleton
Source: Dr Tobias Vogt

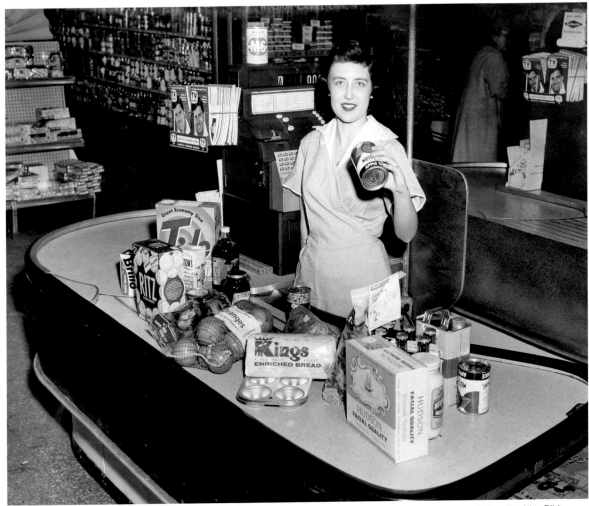

A 1960 photo of a Kings checkout worker is among the items at the New Jersey Supermarket Archives at Rutgers University. Allen Bildner, whose parents founded Kings in the 1930s, donated memorabilia from the chain's early days.
Source: Special Collections and University Archives, Rutgers University Libraries

Hidden hunger in the developed world

Hidden hunger, also known as chronic micronutrient malnutrition, is experienced by more than one in three of the world's total population. This term refers to a chronic lack of vitamins and minerals, which is not immediately apparent and which can exist for a long time before clinical signs of malnutrition become obvious.

It is a popular perception that most people who live in the developed countries of the world enjoy a nutritionally sound diet and are not prey to hidden hunger. The reality is, however, different. Micronutrient inadequacies are to be found in the developed world as well as in the developing world, and their current rate of growth in the developed world gives cause for concern. Growing evidence from

intake surveys in Western countries such as the USA, Canada, Germany, France, Great Britain and many others indicates that a sufficient intake is not being achieved in the case of some micronutrients, according to recommendations using RDAs as reference. This is especially the case for folic acid, vitamin D, vitamin E, iron and iodine.

According to the United Nations Food and Agriculture Organization (FAO), micronutrient inadequacies may, in the long term, lead to a wide number of health problems, including impaired cognitive development, lower resistance to disease, and increased risks during childbirth for both mothers and children. A particular issue in the developed world is the inadequate folic acid intake and vitamin D status.

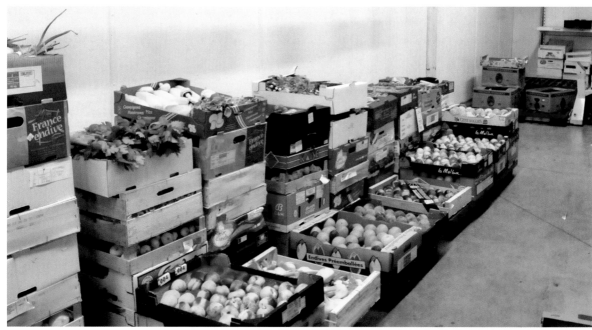

Food bank in Hérault, France: The growth of food banks in the developed world is a sign that nutrition insecurity is by no means confined to the developing world.
Source: Anne-Catherine Frey

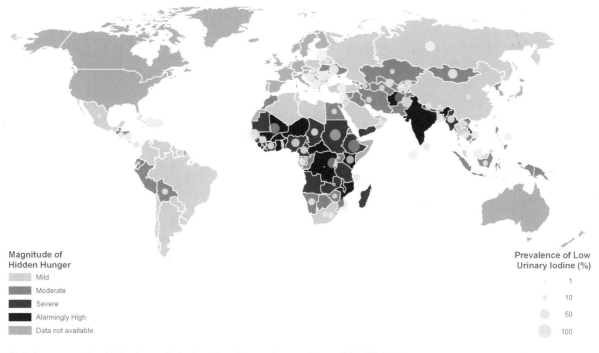

Magnitude of Hidden Hunger
- Mild
- Moderate
- Severe
- Alarmingly High
- Data not available

Prevalence of Low Urinary Iodine (%)
- 1
- 10
- 50
- 100

Global map presenting hidden hunger index based on the prevalence estimates (HHI-PD) in 149 countries and prevalence of low urinary iodine concentration in 90 countries with 2007 Human Development Index <0.9.
The hidden hunger index HHI-PD was estimated based on national estimates of the prevalence of stunting, anemia due to iron deficiency, and low serum retinol concentration.
Source: doi:10.1371/journal.pone.0067860.g002

43 Key definitions

Macronutrient deficiency

This type of malnutrition, known as Protein Energy Malnutrition (PEM), involves a lack of protein and food containing enough calories. This term is applied when hunger is defined in terms of an insufficient intake of calories.

Micronutrient deficiency

Unlike PEM, persons suffering from this type of deficiency may display no outward signs or symptoms. As long as no significant clinical symptoms appear, no consideration is given to the possibility of a micronutrient deficiency. This begs the question of whether a shortfall of the recommended dietary allowances (RDA) is pathologically significant and, if so, how a diagnosis can be made.

Common micronutrient deficiencies

The most common micronutrient deficiencies among women and children are lack of iodine, which is essential for bodily and mental development; iron, a lack of which causes anemia and hampers the cognitive development of children; and vitamin A, which is needed for healthy eyesight and a healthy immune system.

It is often overlooked that behind each of the deficiencies attributed by UNICEF to an unbalanced diet there exist further deficiencies that are not yet visible, yet which exert a negative impact on a child's development. Likewise, a lack of other micronutrients than the above-mentioned three can hamper development long before symptoms are apparent.

The fact that both the FAO and the WHO define hunger in purely quantitative terms – i.e., the result of too few calories – misses the mark. Even if the subjective aspect of hunger, the empty feeling in one's stomach, is addressed by this definition, there is another aspect of hunger which is left out: the body's craving for essential nutritional components. This is what is meant by 'hidden hunger'.

Dimensions of hidden hunger

The human body extracts 51 different essential compounds from food which it cannot produce itself through metabolism. Among these, as far as we currently know, are amino acids, as well as so-called micronutrients (vitamins, trace elements and minerals), which exert a direct influence on physical and mental development and the immune system, and are vital to the body's metabolic processes. To date, it is only known what effects the lack of a certain few micronutrients have on the body in the form of clinical symptoms, such as scurvy (due to a lack of vitamin C), rickets (caused by a vitamin D deficiency), beriberi (triggered by too little vitamin B) and pellagra (resulting from niacin deficiency). This naturally does not exclude the possibility that the micronutrients which have hitherto been the object of less analysis also have an impact on our susceptibility to certain illnesses or the onset of such ailments later in life.

The consequences of a micronutrient deficiency

Both sides of the coin – the causes and adverse effects of the above-mentioned micronutrient deficiencies – are nothing new and have been researched at length. It is therefore quite astounding that they are not considered when assessing the food situation in the world. Moreover, the 'hidden' deficits of micronutrient deficiencies are known, and recommendations are given to avoid a deficiency, for instance by means of supplements or food fortification. However, it is often overlooked that the underlying cause of such deficiencies is a diet which does not meet the nutritional needs of most people, not to mention children and pregnant women. It is also not enough to push for a diet which contains all micronutrients, except in cases of acute, life-saving intervention. Hidden hunger must first and foremost be uncovered and then avoided by all means. The negative, in fact devastating, effects of hidden hunger, cannot be reversed once the damage is done.

Source: Hans Konrad Biesalski, Hidden Hunger, Springer-Verlag, Berlin Heidelberg 2013

The return of rickets

Leading doctors [in the UK] are calling for vitamin D supplements to be made more widely available to children to beat the returning scourge of rickets.

Cases of rickets have gone up four-fold in the past 15 years because many pregnant women and young children are not getting enough of the sunshine vitamin.

Says Professor Mitch Blair of the Royal College of Pediatrics and Child Health (RCPCH): "We know vitamin D deficiency is a growing problem, and localized research reveals startlingly high levels of vitamin deficiency among certain groups including children. People can only get a fraction – just 10 percent – of their recommended daily amount of vitamin D through food, and very little from sunlight. So getting out in the sun more or eating more oily fish isn't going to solve the problem."

Lack of vitamin D is related to a plethora of serious illnesses in children and adults that could be prevented through relatively simple steps such as taking supplements.

Diabetes, asthma, multiple sclerosis, tuberculosis, and life-threatening heart disease have been linked to low levels of vitamin D in early life. The RCPCH estimates at least half of the UK's white population, up to 90 percent of the multi-ethnic population and a quarter of children have vitamin D deficiency.

Many people thought rickets had virtually been eliminated after the war, but there has been a recent rise in numbers of children with the disease. Cases went up from 183 in 1995/96 to 762 last year.

Source: Abridged from Return of rickets: Cases up four-fold in the last 15 years as pregnant women and children fail to get enough Vitamin D. Jenny Hope, Mail Online, December 14 2012.

An increase in poverty and poor nutrition in the developed world

An increase in poverty in industrialized countries, with children primarily affected, is an issue that is often overlooked. Being poor means having a poor diet and little dietary diversity in many cases, which means that children who live in the land of plenty may also suffer from malnutrition. Sadly, this fact seems to interest only a very few people.

In a recent article in the Financial Times magazine, Where austerity really hits home, Gillian Tett raises the issue of hunger in the United Kingdom, with an example from a deprived area of Liverpool:

"There's a lot of little kids going hungry round here," explained one friend, who works in a local community center. Indeed, just the other day she had spoken to a family where the child had been chewing wallpaper at night. "He didn't want to tell his mum because he knew she didn't have the money for supper," she explained. "We hear more and more stories like this."

Gillian Tett's anecdotal evidence of poverty and hunger as a growing problem is backed by figures from the Trussell Trust, providers of a network of food banks around the UK, who state:

"In 2011–12 food banks fed 128,687 people nationwide, in 2012–13 we anticipate this number will rise to over 290,000. Rising costs of food and fuel combined with static income, high unemployment and changes to benefits are causing more and more people to come to food banks for help."

The UK is not alone. In Germany, Nanette Ströbele-Benschop and Peter Tinnemann in their paper *Health Inequalities in Berlin, Germany – analysis of local efforts to support socio-economically disadvantaged people* cite a project supported by the Berliner Tafel e.V. to distribute fresh produce on a weekly basis to the most socioeconomically disadvantaged people, which found that the daily number of people served increased by 9% from May 2006 to May 2010.

Source: The Financial Times, March 8, 2013; http://www.ft.com/cms/s/2/7de158e8-86bd-11e2-b907-00144feabdc0.html#axzz2Z7CZFGe8

Child poverty and malnutrition in the US

Child poverty in the US has reached record levels, with almost 17 million children now affected. A growing number are also going hungry on a daily basis. Currently, 47 million Americans are thought to depend on food banks. One in five children receives food aid. For some families, cheap and easy to prepare food can mean unhealthy choices like pizza – increasing the likelihood of obesity and health problems later in life.

In many areas schools take part in a "backpack" program, set up to deliver food parcels to the most vulnerable on a Friday – so that they have enough to eat over the weekend. In eastern Iowa and western Illinois, the River Bend Foodbank now helps 1,500 children in 30 schools through one such scheme. It has seen the numbers needing help rise sharply.

"It's changed dramatically since the recession. We're up about 30% to 40% in terms of the number of people coming forward," says Caren Laughlin, who has worked with food banks for 30 years. "That's not only because so many people have lost their jobs, it's also because the jobs that are replacing them are low paying. You cannot feed a family."

The problems are reflected across America, says the nationwide charity Feeding America, which operates 200 food banks and feeds 37 million people each year, including 14 million children.

It says that, in total, nearly 17 million US children live in homes where getting enough healthy food is not something they can count on.

Source: Abridged from The children going hungry in America, Duncan Walker, BBC News, March 6, 2013

The history of the balanced diet

The pioneering biochemists of the first half of the 20th century revolutionized our understanding of the role that nutrients play in our health. Founders of the new science of nutrition such as Casimir Funk and Tadeusz Reichstein identified and isolated individual vitamins for the first time, and began to map out their complex functioning in the metabolism. A growing appreciation of the essential health-giving properties of these micronutrients led to the concept of the 'balanced diet' which provided adequate levels of proteins, fats and carbohydrates as well as sufficient amounts of vitamins and minerals. Public health policy – intensified by wartime food rationing and underpinned by educational propaganda – promoted the concept of the balanced diet. Despite the privations of war, the population of the United Kingdom, for instance, ate a healthier diet than at any time in history during World War II and the years immediately following. This generation has shown remarkable health and longevity, which are to a great extent traceable to good dietary habits over a long period of time.

The decline of the balanced diet

There is a polarization in dietary lifestyles in the developed world. While the more affluent and educated have the resources to support a healthier lifestyle and diet, those who are economically poor, who live in 'food deserts' and who do not possess a good knowledge of nutrition often do not have access to or cannot afford a healthy, balanced diet or do not have the means to make the right choices. Ironically, the polarization of diets in the developed world has been accompanied by a massive rise in the popularity of cult restaurants and TV chefs.

Sir Jack Cecil Drummond: A pioneer of nutrition science

Sir Jack Cecil Drummond was a Professor of Biochemistry who isolated pure vitamin A in the 1930s, but perhaps his greatest achievements were in translating original science into practical dietary programs. His obituary in the *British Journal of Nutrition* in 1954 praised these efforts:

"Perhaps Drummond's name is most closely associated with the provision of special foods for mothers and children. From the outset he pressed the claims of nutritionally vulnerable groups. The success of his efforts in this direction is seen in the schemes that were gradually evolved for the cheap supply and priority rationing of liquid milk, in the early experiments with blackcurrant syrup and rosehip syrup as sources of vitamins for expectant mothers and young children, in the subsequent provision of concentrated orange juice and cod-liver oil to these two groups, and in the generous allocation of rationed foods for school meals and the provision of national milk cocoa for adolescents."

Drummond developed a system of national rationing to ensure that everyone, whether rich or poor, had an adequate nutritional intake. As James Fergusson writes in his 2007 publication *The Vitamin Murders*:

"The health of the British nation, schoolchildren included, was not just maintained during the Second World War but improved...[T]he incidence of almost every diet-related illness was lower than it had ever been. Drummond was a genuine home-front hero."

As Tom Jaine writes in his introduction to the 1991 edition of Drummond's *The Englishman's Food: Five Centuries of English Diet*:

Drummond was working during the heroic period of nutritional science when the constituents of food necessary to maintain, and then improve, the quality of life were finally defined. This... was the era when deficiency diseases received their full investigation. For centuries rickets, scurvy, pellagra, beri-beri, night blindness and hunger-oedema had been the scourge of various societies...but it needed the new nutrition to fully explain the treatment and to rapidly extend the benefits of cure to as many populations as possible."

Source: Abridged from Sir Jack Cecil Drummond DSc, FRIC, FRS: A hero of nutrition science and advocacy by Jonathan Steffen, Sight and Life 2/2012

'Food deserts' and the problem of limited access to balanced nutrition

The more varied one's diet is, the healthier it is. Normal body weight and growth can only be achieved if children take their food from several different sources.

Dietary diversity depends upon certain factors, for instance that different foods are available and also affordable. It is this lack of diversity that is responsible for malnutrition and all of its harmful consequences.

There are districts in both urban environments and rural settings, where shops do not stock the range of fresh and nutritious foods necessary for a balanced diet. These areas are usually characterized by convenience stores that stock only processed foods and by fast-food restaurants. Residents who are unable, for whatever reason, to travel further afield in search of a better diet therefore find themselves in a situation where there is food to buy but the nutritional value of that food is inadequate.

In 2010 the United States Department of Agriculture defined what's considered a 'food desert' as follows: "To qualify as a 'low-access community,' at least 500 people and/or at least 33 percent of the census tract's population must reside more than one mile from a supermarket or large grocery store (for rural census tracts, the distance is more than 10 miles)."

Food deserts in the US and other barriers to a balanced diet

The United States Department of Agriculture (USDA) has replaced their original *Food Desert Locator* with the more detailed *Food Access Research Atlas*. This sophisticated mapping tool allows users to investigate multiple indicators of food store access, and highlights the areas of the US which can be classified as 'food deserts'

It should be pointed out that, in all cultural and geographical settings, the question of access to food has many dimensions, and that a variety of factors may combine to prevent an individual, or a group of individuals, from enjoying a balanced diet. These may include, for instance, lack of mobility (lack of transport or lack of physical mobility due to illness or infirmity), lack of purchasing power, and also a lack of understanding of basic nutritional principles. Within the world's most affluent societies, there are individuals – whether in hospitals, care homes or hospices, whether in substandard housing or sleeping rough in the street, who do not have access to that 'simplest' thing, a healthy, balanced diet.

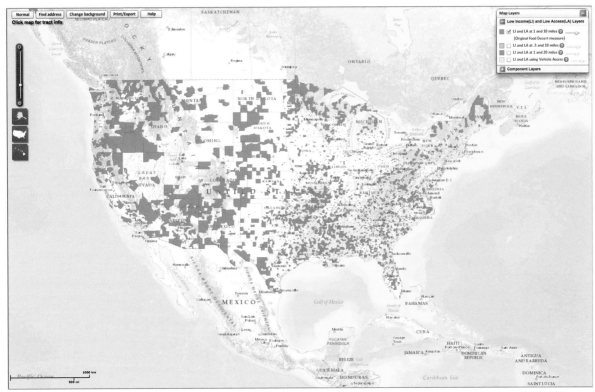

Screenshot from the USDA's 'Food Access Research Atlas', showing food deserts in the US
Source: http://www.ers.usda.gov/data-products/food-access-research-atlas.aspx#.UVBiGELd7dk

The long-term consequences of inadequate nutrition

The long-term consequences of malnutrition and hidden hunger in the developed world are significant. For example inadequate and suboptimal vitamin D status alone is known to be a risk factor for some cancers such as breast cancer, prostate cancer, and several autoimmune diseases such as multiple sclerosis, rheumatoid arthritis and type-1 diabetes. An unhealthy, unbalanced diet rich in unsaturated fats, sugars and salts may contribute to a wide range of non-communicable diseases such as cardiovascular diseases, cancers, chronic respiratory diseases and diabetes.

In September 2011 the United Nations launched an effort to tackle non-communicable diseases (NCDs) such as cancer and diabetes with a summit meeting devoted to curbing the factors, such as tobacco and alcohol use behind the often-preventable scourge that causes 63 percent of all deaths. The two-day high-level General Assembly meeting adopted a declaration calling for a multi-pronged campaign by governments, industry and civil society to set up by 2013 the plans needed to curb the risk factors behind the four

groups of NCDs – cardiovascular diseases, cancers, chronic respiratory diseases and diabetes.

As well as steps to curb the use of tobacco and alcohol, the UN advocated steps to curb "the extensive marketing to children, particularly on television, of foods and beverages that are high in saturated fats, trans-fatty acids, sugars, or salt."

Vitamin D has important benefits in lowering the risk of fractures, improving muscle strength, and reducing the risk of a number of conditions and diseases. The benefit regarding the reduction of fractures and the contribution to muscle strength is well reported, while other benefits are still emerging, covering areas such as type 2 diabetes, cardiovascular disease, some types of cancers, strengthening of the immune system, and autoimmune diseases such as multiple sclerosis.[1,2]

Many people have a low level of serum vitamin D (measured as 25-hydroxy-vitamin D) owing to poor access to natural sources of vitamin D. This may be attributable, for instance, to factors such as an absence of cold-water ocean fish from the diet, living largely indoors and therefore getting insufficient exposure to sunlight, and inhabiting the high latitudes of the world. The reduction of the direct and indirect costs associated with the above-mentioned diseases is based on randomized controlled trials using an intake of 200–800 IU vitamin D, which results in an adequate vitamin D status.

Assessments by various research groups indicate that the financial burden on direct and indirect healthcare costs arising from inadequate micronutrient status in the

developed world could be in the range of billions of euros.[3]

Economics aside it is, above all, a question of humanity. If we took the rights of every individual to an adequate diet as seriously as we take the issue of human rights, and if we proclaimed these as loudly and often as we rightly do with regard to human rights, then the first big step toward making a change would be taken.

Hidden hunger across the life cycle

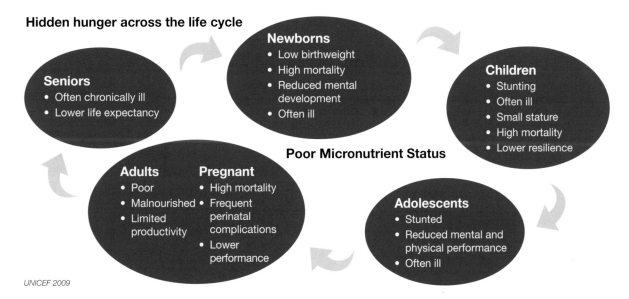

Newborns
• Low birthweight
• High mortality
• Reduced mental development
• Often ill

Children
• Stunting
• Often ill
• Small stature
• High mortality
• Lower resilience

Seniors
• Often chronically ill
• Lower life expectancy

Poor Micronutrient Status

Adults
• Poor
• Malnourished
• Limited productivity

Pregnant
• High mortality
• Frequent perinatal complications
• Lower performance

Adolescents
• Stunted
• Reduced mental and physical performance
• Often ill

UNICEF 2009

The economic impact of vitamin D deficiency

In developed countries, at least 10% of people in the general population and up to 70% and more of individuals in specific patient groups have blood vitamin D levels lying in the deficiency range (e.g. 25- hydroxy vitamin D levels <30 nmol/L). Vitamin D deficiency is probably the most frequent micronutrient deficiency in developed countries. In westernized societies, the economic burden of the healthcare system is high and will further increase in future due to demographic changes and the increasing proportion of elderly people.

In Europe, total expenditure on health varies between 6% (Eastern Europe) and more than 11% (Western Europe) of gross domestic product. Thus, an estimated annual amount of one trillion euros is spent on the healthcare system in Europe. A recent meta-analysis of pooled patient-level data from randomized controlled

trials provided convincing evidence that between 14% and 30% of nonvertebral fractures can be prevented by adequate vitamin D supply. Based on these data it can be calculated that in Europe alone, fracture prevention by supplementary vitamin D would result in cost savings of approximately five billion euros. There is some evidence from genetic studies, prospective cohort studies and randomized controlled trials that vitamin D may play a role in the prevention of type 1 diabetes, infections and cardiovascular-related deaths. Vitamin D may also reduce the risk of exacerbations in patients with chronic obstructive pulmonary disease and multiple sclerosis. Although there is much uncertainty about the cost savings potential of adequate vitamin D supply, the amount may reach the binary billions range.

Source: Abridged from Economic impact of undernutrition: Vitamin D by A. Zittermann, University Bochum and Bad Oeynhausen

Annual income and diet cost comparison

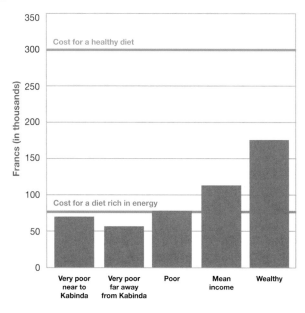

Save the Children 2010

Undernourished persons (in millions)

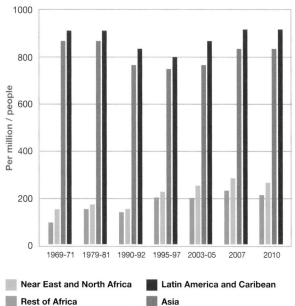

Fischer et al. 2008; input from FAOSTAT.fao.org 2011, 2012

Trapped in the cycle of hunger, generation after generation

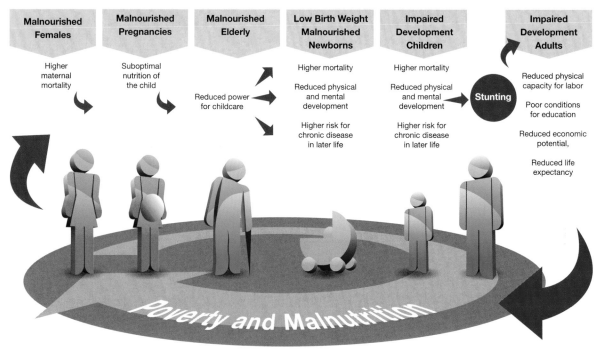

Modified from: ACC/SCN 2000

My personal view

Hans Konrad Biesalski
Head of the Department of Biological Chemistry and Nutrition, University of Hohenheim, Stuttgart, Germany

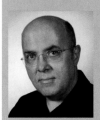

We have clear evidence that income is related to food security, and we have a range of data showing that a balanced diet is related to higher income and higher education.

We need to evaluate food security, in particular in females and young children living in poverty, because inadequacy of micronutrient supply during the short time period of the 1,000-day window may also in developed countries have an impact on further development and consequently on the economic and health future of the child.

It may be that the magnitude of this problem is overestimated in the developed world. Nevertheless, as long as we lack data of sufficient quality on this subject, this problem should concern us. Nutrition science is based on molecular biology on the one hand and on research related to obesity on the other. Both have an excellent economically driven lobby. Malnutrition, however, is not in the focus of nutrition scientists, even though its impact is as serious as is that of overnutrition.

Further reading

Biesalski, HK. Hidden Hunger. Berlin/Heidelberg, Germany: Springer-Verlag, 2013.

Roman Vinas B, Ribas Barba L, Ngo J. Projected prevalence of inadequate nutrient intakes in Europe. Ann Nutr Metab 2011;59:84-95.

Wahl DA, Cooper C, Ebeling PR et al. A global representation of vitamin D status in healthy populations. Arch Osteoporos, 2012;7(1–2):155-172.

Bailey RL, Dodd KW, Gahche JJ et al. Total folate and folic acid intake from foods and dietary supplements in the United States: 2003–2006. Am J Clin Nutr 2010;91:231–237.

Bischoff-Ferrari HA, Willet WC, Orav EJ et al. A pooled analysis of vitamin D dose requirements for fracture prevention. NEJM 2012;367:40–49.

Flynn A, Hirvonen T, Mensink GB et al. Intake of selected nutrients from foods, from fortification and from supplements in various European countries. Food Nutr Res 2009;53:1–51.

Bischoff-Ferrari H. Health effects of vitamin D. Dermatol Ther 2010;23(1):23–30.

Fulgoni VL, Keast DR, Bailey RL et al. Foods, fortificants, and supplements: where do Americans get their nutrients? J Nutr 2011;141:1847–1854.

Grant WB, Cross HS, Garland CF et al. Estimated benefit of increased vitamin D status in reducing the economic burden of disease in Europe. Prog Biophys Mol Biol 2009;99:104–113.

Zittermann A, Kuhn J, Dreier J. Vitamin D status and the risk of major adverse cardiac and cerebrovascular events in cardiac surgery. Eur Heart J 2013;34(18):1358–64.

Zittermann A. The estimated benefits of vitamin D for Germany. Mol Nutr Food Res 2010;54(8):1164–71.

Chapter Four

The Obesity Crisis

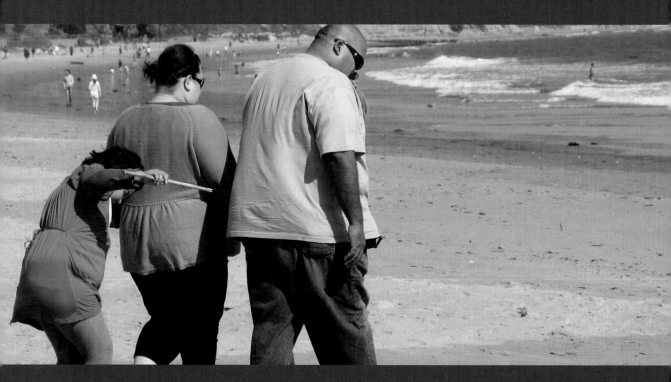

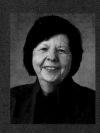

Eileen Kennedy

Professor of Nutrition,
Former Dean of the Friedman School of Nutrition Science and Policy,
Tufts University, Boston, USA

"The rise of childhood obesity has placed the health of an entire generation at risk."

Tom Vilsack, United States Secretary of Agriculture

Key messages

- The current increase in obesity in the global population is unprecedented.

- Worldwide, approximately 1.4 billion adults are overweight, and 500 million are obese.

- As the most common cause of death, infectious diseases have now been overtaken by non-communicable diseases (NCDs).

- In many low-income countries wealthy and well-educated people are more likely to be overweight than the poor.

- In higher-income countries lower-income populations tend to be more at risk of obesity and its long-term consequences. policy-makers in developing countries need to pay greater attention to the obesity crisis and its linkages to undernutrition.

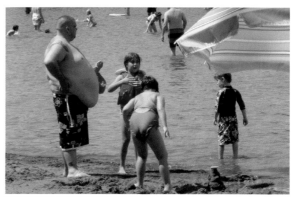

The problem of obesity has assumed epidemic proportions in recent years
Source: Sight and Life

The world continues to experience malnutrition and undernutrition on an unprecedented scale. So huge and complex is this problem that it sometimes diverts attention from another rapidly growing issue which has vast ramifications and will have severe long-term consequences: the rise of obesity.

According to the United Nations World Health Organization (WHO), 1.4 billion adults worldwide are overweight, and of these, approximately 300 million women and 200 million men are obese. Worldwide obesity has doubled since 1980, in fact, and 65% of the world's population now lives in countries where overweight and obesity related diseases kill more people than undernutrition.

This is a dramatic reversal of the traditional paradigm whereby poor diet is associated exclusively with undernutrition. What makes it especially concerning is the fact that overweight and obesity can lead to health problems such as diabetes, hypertension, heart disease and cancer. The significant increase in the prevalence of these non-communicable diseases (NCDs) in recent years is directly attributable to the rise in obesity in the world's population. The traditional focus of governments and NGOs on eliminating starvation and hunger, however, tends to divert attention from this growing public health problem. It is hard to imagine that a person can overeat their way to malnutrition. But this is precisely what is happening.

53

The nutrition transition

In poorer regions of the world and poorer sections of society in general, the staple diet has traditionally been low in fat, generally taking the form of cereals and pulses and being supplemented as and when possible by nutrient-rich animal protein. The past few decades have witnessed a 'nutrition transition' to a more Western-influenced diet in many parts of the globe, however. This diet offers more diversity, but contains considerably more saturated fats, total fats, sugars, starches and animal proteins.

A striking example of this phenomenon is to be found in Micronesia in the Pacific Ocean. According to the Bulletin of the World Health Organization (Volume 88, Number 7, July 2010, 481–560), "Replacing traditional foods with imported, processed food has contributed to the high prevalence of obesity and related health problems in the Pacific Islands ... Beyond the image of white sandy beaches and carefree lifestyles, the Pacific Islands are facing serious health problems, the prime culprit being imported foods. In at least 10 Pacific Islands more than 50% (and in some, up to 90%) of the population is overweight ... Obesity prevalence ranges from more than 30% in Fiji to a staggering 80% among women in American Samoa, a territory of the United States of America (USA). WHO defines overweight as having a body mass index (BMI) equal to or more than 25, and obesity as a BMI equal to or more than 30. Diabetes prevalence among adults in the Pacific region is among the highest in the world; 47% in American Samoa compared with 13% in mainland USA, and it ranges from 14% to 44% elsewhere in the region."

Stranger than paradise

Micronutrient deficiencies are common in the Pacific Islands. In 15 of 16 countries surveyed, more than one fifth of children and pregnant women were anemic. In Fiji, Papua New Guinea and Vanuatu, iodine deficiency and related goiter are endemic. Vitamin A deficiency is also a significant public health risk in Kiribati, the Marshall Islands, the Federated States of Micronesia and Papua New Guinea.

About 40% of the Pacific Island region's population of 9.7 million has been diagnosed with a NCD, notably cardiovascular disease, diabetes and hypertension. These diseases account for three quarters of all deaths across the Pacific archipelago and 40–60% of total healthcare expenditure, according to a meeting on obesity prevention and control strategies in the Pacific held in Samoa in September 2000.

Dr Temo K Waqanivalu, technical officer for nutrition and physical activity at the Office of the WHO Representative for the South Pacific in Suva, Fiji, partly blames poor diet for the region's health problems. "Promotion of traditional foods has fallen by the wayside. They are unable to compete with the glamour and flashiness of imported foods," he says.

People in the Pacific Islands may know what constitutes healthy eating but, as in many parts of the world, governments struggle to change people's behavior. In eight countries, less than 20% of people surveyed reported eating the recommended five or more portions of fruit and vegetables a day. The often calorie-rich and nutrient-poor imported foods have a stronger appeal.

Life expectancy data make clear the urgent need for action. The average age at which people develop diabetes and cardiovascular disease is getting lower. In Fiji, only 16% of the population is aged more than 55 years due to premature deaths primarily caused by non-communicable diseases.

Source: Bulletin of the World Health Organization (Volume 88, Number 7, July 2010, 481–560)

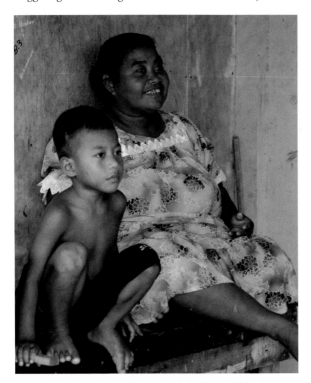

The double burden of malnutrition: parental obesity and child malnutrition often exist side by side
Source: Sight and Life

The extremes witnessed among the populations of the Pacific Islands are part of a trend that is leaving no corner of the globe unaffected. Certain populations – inhabitants of the Indian subcontinent, for instance, or the Pima Indians in the United States – are especially susceptible to weight gain in the face of exposure to a Western diet rich in fats, sugars and starches. But the whole world is affected by the general trend towards a more sedentary lifestyle. Whereas before World War II, the majority of the world's population worked in agriculture, manufacturing or some other area requiring physical effort, the proliferation of labor-saving devices, automotive transportation and computerization has vastly and rapidly reduced the need to expend physical effort during the course of a normal day. People are burning off fewer calories during their day-to-day lives and at the same time consuming more calories. This inevitably results in weight gain. The combination of a change in dietary patterns plus a change in lifestyle has brought about the simple formula for obesity: 'energy in' exceeds 'energy out'.

According to the Morbidity and Mortality Report published in 2004 by the Centers for Disease Control and Prevention, in 1971, women in the US consumed an average of 1,542 calories per day compared with 1,877 in 2004. Men consumed an average of 2,450 calories in 1971, but consumed an average of 2,616 calories in 2004. So in a time frame of just over 30 years, average calorie intake increased by 22% for women, and 10% for men. It is not surprising then, that obesity has become a major problem in the US.

Unless people compensate for increased calorie intake by means of increased energy expenditure, they will put on unnecessary weight.

The United States and Western Europe were the first regions of the world to go through the nutrition transition. In the 1920s and 1930s, during the Great Depression, these regions contained many food-insecure people and households. By the 1950s and 1960s, greater affluence led to richer diets, with an evening meal usually comprising meat, potatoes and vegetables for even the poorer sections of society. This did not lead to obesity on a wide scale, however, for the fast-food culture of today was still in its infancy and lifestyles were still comparatively active for most people. The situation has changed radically in recent years in the US, however, with a knock-on effect that extends beyond the shores of the United States and to the furthest corners of the globe.

The poorest countries of the world are now going through the nutrition transition first charted by America, and they too have seen an increase in the proportion of the population that is overweight and obese. This increase has been followed by a dramatic increase in non-communicable diseases, particularly type 2 diabetes. Recent statistics from the World Health Organization show that 44% of the world diabetes burden, 23% of the ischemic heart disease burden and between 7% and 41% of certain cancer burdens are attributable to overweight and obesity.

Definitions of key terms

Overweight for adults is a BMI between 25 and 29.99

Obesity for adults is a BMI 30 to 39.99

Morbidly obese for adults is BMI 40 or greater

Note: BMI is weight (kg)/height squared (meters)

For children, overweight is 85th to 95th percentile on child growth chart, and obesity is more than the 95%

Type 1 diabetes, also sometimes called juvenile-onset diabetes or insulin-dependent diabetes is a chronic condition in which the pancreas produces little or no insulin.

Type 2 diabetes, also sometimes called adult-onset or non-insulin-dependent diabetes, is a chronic condition that affects the way the body metabolizes sugars. With type 2 diabetes, the body either resists the effects of insulin or else

does not produce enough insulin.

"Diabesity" is a term coined by Dr Francine Kaufman to indicate a combination of diabetes and obesity.

Non-communicable diseases (NCDs) – also known as chronic diseases – are not transmitted from person to person. NCDs can progress slowly and persist in the body for decades. The main types of NCDs include cardiovascular disease, cancers, respiratory diseases and diabetes.

"Hidden hunger" is another name for micronutrient malnutrition. This term is used since the specific deficiency is typically not visible.

The "double burden of malnutrition" is defined as the coexistence of undernutrition and overweight in the same community or even the same household.

Case study

The Pima Indians: A case study of the relationship between obesity and diabetes

The National Institute of Diabetes and Digestive and Kidney Diseases (NIDDK)

Research conducted on the Pima Indians for the past 30 years has helped scientists prove that obesity is a major risk factor in the development of diabetes. One half of adult Pima Indians have diabetes and 95% of those with diabetes are overweight.

These studies, carried out with the help of the Pima Indians, have shown that before gaining weight, overweight people have a slower metabolic rate compared to people of the same weight. This slower metabolic rate, combined with a high-fat diet and a genetic tendency to retain fat may cause the epidemic overweight seen in the Pima Indians, scientists believe.

Along with genetic make-up, diet is a key factor to healthy lifestyle. The influence of traditional desert crops on the metabolism of the Pima Indians is being studied to determine how to prevent the onset of diabetes and obesity.

Scientists use the "thrifty gene" theory proposed in 1962 by geneticist James Neel to help explain why many Pima Indians are overweight. Neel's theory is based on the fact that for thousands of years populations who relied on farming, hunting and fishing for food, such as the Pima Indians, experienced alternating periods of feast and famine. Neel said that to adapt to these extreme changes in caloric needs, these people developed a thrifty gene that allowed them to store fat during times of plenty so that they would not starve during times of famine.

This gene was helpful as long as there were periods of famine. But once these populations adopted the typical Western lifestyle, with less physical activity, a high-fat diet, and access to a constant supply of calories, this gene began to work against them, continuing to store calories in preparation for famine. Scientists think that the thrifty gene that once protected people from starvation might also contribute to their retaining unhealthy amounts of fat.

There are approximately 100,000 genes packed into 23 pairs of chromosomes in every cell of a person's body. Within a gene, chemicals form individual codes, like words, which tell the cells of the body what to do. It is the code within a gene that directs the body to grow skin, and determines whether the skin is brown, yellow, black or white; to form hair and bone; to circulate blood and hormones such as adrenalin and insulin; and to perform every other biological process in the body.

Some diseases are caused by bacteria or viruses that infect the body and make it sick. Others, such as diabetes, occur because a gene's code causes it to function differently under some circumstances. For instance, if a person has a gene that makes that person likely to get diabetes, eating a lot of high-fat food over time may increase that person's chance of getting sick. On the other hand, eating lower fat foods such as fruits and vegetables and exercising each day may help to prevent the disease. A person can't choose his or her genes, but can choose what to eat and whether or not to exercise.

Finding the gene or genes that may increase a person's risk for getting diabetes and obesity is the most effective way scientists have to learn what's wrong in a diabetic person.

With the help of the Pima Indians, National Institutes of Health (NIH) scientists have already learned that diabetes develops when a person's body doesn't use insulin effectively. They know that other genes probably influence some people's bodies to burn energy at a slow rate, and/or to want to eat more, making it more likely that they will become overweight. Being overweight, in turn, puts a person at even higher risk for diabetes. Because they have learned this over 30 years of working with the Pima Indians, NIH scientists now are able to test ways to prevent the disease with low-fat diets and regular exercise.

Source: http://diabetes.niddk.nih.gov/dm/pubs/pima/obesity/obesity.htm, March 2013

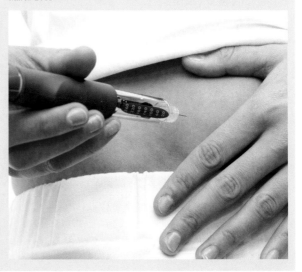

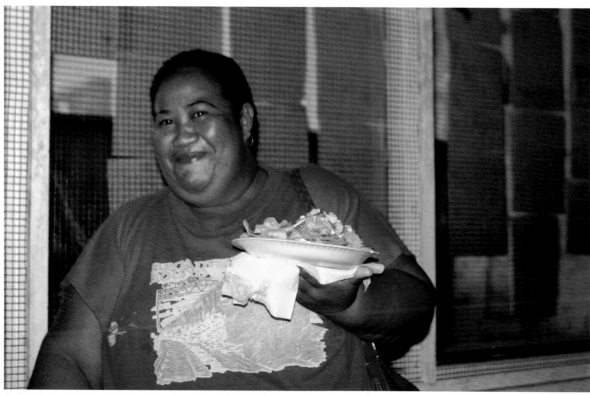

An inhabitant of Pohnpei in Micronesia, where diet-related obesity is a problem of epidemic proportions
Source: Sight and Life

The critical first one thousand days

The Scaling Up Nutrition (SUN) Movement was launched in September 2010. The SUN Movement stresses direct nutrition interventions of known efficacy targeted to pregnant women and children up to age two. The direct nutrition interventions are complemented by nutrition-sensitive policies and programs. SUN addresses undernutrition; ironically, by improving nutritional status in the first 1,000 days, health and nutrition in adulthood can be enhanced. The developmental origins of health and disease (DOHaD), also called the Barker Hypothesis, uncovered a relationship between birth weight and chronic disease. Infants born small have a higher risk of obesity, hypertension, coronary heart disease and diabetes. Environmental stresses, primarily in utero, alter structures of organs and change regulatory gene expression, resulting in an increased risk of chronic disease later in life. Thus, poor maternal diet has a double, negative effect of contributing to a lower birth weight, an increased risk of developmental disorders and higher risk of chronic disease later in life. Effective nutrition interventions aimed at the 1,000 days have immediate as well as long-term health consequences.

The time bomb of obesity

In the past few years, non-communicable diseases such as heart disease, diabetes and cancer have overtaken infectious diseases as the major cause of death globally. However, health policy in developing countries still tends to focus on combating undernutrition and infectious diseases only, rather than tackling the obesity epidemic and its consequences at the same time. There is a general perception that if people are overweight, then they have more than enough food and are not in need of help. The time bomb of NCDs linked to obesity is all too frequently overlooked. The Millennium Development Goals, for example, do not include a goal related to NCDs.

According to WHO, many low- and middle-income countries are now facing a "double burden" of disease. While they continue to deal with the problems of infectious disease and undernutrition, they are experiencing a rapid upsurge in non-communicable disease risk factors such as obesity and overweight, particularly in urban settings. It is not uncommon to find undernutrition and obesity existing side by side within the same country, the same community and even the same household.

The double burden of malnutrition

Many developing countries now face the double burden of malnutrition, defined as the coexistence of undernutrition and overweight in the same community or even in the same household.

This study sought to estimate the prevalence of the double burden of malnutrition and to identify associated maternal, child, and household characteristics in rural Indonesia and Bangladesh.

A total of 247,126 rural households that participated in the Indonesia Nutrition Surveillance System (2000–2003) and 168,317 rural households in the Bangladesh Nutritional Surveillance Project (2003–2006) were included in the analysis. Maternal and child double burden (MCDB) and its association with individual and household characteristics were determined by using logistic regression models.

MCDB was observed in 11% and 4% of the households in rural Indonesia and Bangladesh, respectively. Maternal short stature, and older age of mothers were strong predictors of MCDB. Child characteristics such as older age and being female were associated with an increased risk of MCDB, whereas currently being breastfed was protective against MCDB. A large family size and higher weekly per capita household expenditure was a strong predictor of MCDB.

This study showed for the first time that even in Bangladesh the double burden is not exclusive to urban areas. Therefore, future policies and interventions should address under- and overweight simultaneously in both rural and urban developing country settings.

Source: Oddo VM, Rah JH, Semba RD, Sun K, Akhter N, Sari M, de Pee S, Moench-Pfanner R, Bloem M, Kraemer K. Predictors of maternal and child double burden of malnutrition in rural Indonesia and Bangladesh. Am J Clin Nutr. 2012; 95(4):951–8.

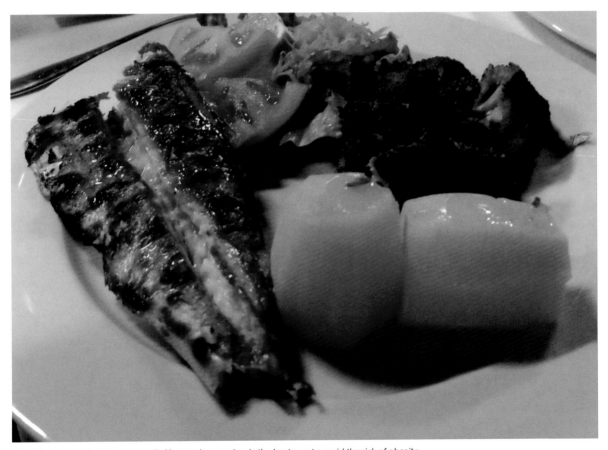

A healthy, balanced diet, accompanied by regular exercise, is the best way to avoid the risk of obesity
Source: Sight and Life

Double Burden of Malnutrition: Time to Drop "Double"?

One of the things that is apparent from the recent Lancet Nutrition Series is that it is becoming more and more difficult to keep the under- and overnutrition agendas separate.

It is really tempting to keep them separate.

First, dealing with undernutrition is difficult enough without having to deal with overnutrition … And of course, dealing with undernutrition is one great way to help prevent overnutrition later in life. In addition, dealing with overnutrition means having to grapple with the food industry and a whole range of factors outside of nutrition's comfort zone: urban development, education, trade, taxes and agriculture for example. Also, there aren't exactly a range of interventions and policies that have been shown to be effective to inspire us to ramp up action on the overnutrition front. Finally, it is not easy to get research funding to address the two in an integrated fashion.

But I think the separation … is no longer sustainable. First, overnutrition does not operate in a different space: it is not just a later in life phenomenon – it is happening to under fives; it is not just in urban areas and it is not just in middle- and upper- income countries – it is everywhere. Second, the undernutrition community can't avoid engaging with the private sector – not having to deal with the private sector is no longer a reason for not getting involved in overnutrition. Third, we now know that the fight against undernutrition has to go way beyond health, and into the wider development space. This is something even more obvious in dealing with overnutriton.

All the reasons for separating the two are dissolving.

So, seemingly, something that is difficult (undernutrition reduction) just got much harder (dealing with under- and overnutrition). But is that really so? Can an integrated approach help us address both issues better? I think that may be the case.

Making development more nutrition-sensitive and making nutrition more politically aware surely brings the worlds of over- and undernutrition together, indeed, shows they were never that far apart in the first place. They should no longer be separated at birth.

In this context, a new review of Global Evidence on the Double Burden of Malnutrition from the World Bank (by Roger Shrimpton and Claudia Rokx) is comprehensive and well done, but depressing … It is depressing because it shows how divided the two camps are and how that is to either's advantage. Beyond the physiological linkages there

has not been much thinking in the past 10 years on how to bring them together in the policy, program, training, communication and advocacy spaces.

Perhaps the time is only now right to do this.

A paper in the Lancet from December 2012 by Moodle et al. ("Profits and Pandemics") draws the parallels between the practices of the tobacco, alcohol and "ultra-processed food and drink" industries. They conclude that "despite the common reliance on industry self-regulation and public-private partnerships, there is no evidence of their effectiveness or safety". I think the evidence base upon which they draw is weak (not their fault), but their conclusions are in accord with my own sense of the situation and indeed I made the same parallels in a Development Policy Review paper from 2003 where I go through the various triggers for successful government regulation of tobacco and see how they apply to obesity.

I think policy-makers are about to get a wakeup call from advocacy groups, consumers, the health community, and even some industry leaders, to do something.

The Double Burden is here to stay. Perhaps it is time to drop the Double (on the double).

Source: Lawrence Haddad, Institute of Development Studies (http://www. developmenthorizons.com/2013/06/double-burden-of-malnutrition-time-to.html? utm_source= feedburner&utm_medium=email&utm_ campaign=Feed %3A+ DevelopmentHorizons+%28Development+Horizons%29) 23 June 2013

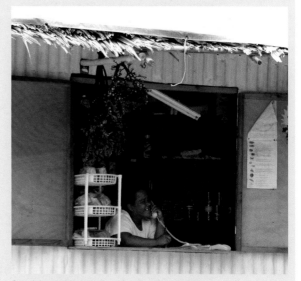

Snack bar in Micronesia with overweight manager
Source: Sight and Life

Childhood obesity

Once considered a high-income country problem, overweight and obesity are now on the rise in low- and middle-income countries, particularly in urban settings. More than 30 million overweight children are living in developing countries and 10 million in developed countries.

Children in low- and middle-income countries are more vulnerable to inadequate prenatal, infant and young child nutrition. At the same time, they are exposed to high-fat, high-sugar, high-salt, energy-dense, micronutrient-poor foods, which tend to be lower in cost but also lower in nutrient quantity and quality. These dietary patterns in conjunction with lower levels of physical activity, result in sharp increases in childhood obesity while undernutrition issues remain unsolved.

Childhood obesity is associated with a higher chance of obesity, premature death and disability in adulthood. But in addition to increased future risks, obese children experience breathing difficulties, increased risk of fractures, hypertension, early markers of cardiovascular disease, insulin resistance and psychological effects.

Source: WHO Fact Sheet 311, March 2013

Protecting children from the negative impact of marketing on dietary behavior

The marketing of food and beverage products high in fat, sugar and salt to children is recognized in Europe as an important element in the etiology of child obesity and in the development of diet-related non-communicable diseases. Overweight is one of the biggest public health challenges of the 21st century: all countries are affected to varying extents, particularly in the lower socioeconomic groups.

The picture is not improving in most countries of the WHO European Region. The figures for children from the WHO Childhood Obesity Surveillance Initiative show that, on average, one child in every three aged 6–9 years is overweight or obese.

The WHO Regional Office for Europe has been working in recent years with Member States to devise policy options that could protect children better from the negative impact of marketing on dietary behavior. This process has been developed by working together in the implementation of the set of recommendations endorsed at the Sixty-third World Health Assembly in 2010 on the marketing of food and non-alcoholic beverages to children, as well as within the context of the WHO European Network on reducing food marketing pressure on children.

The bases of policies to address unacceptable marketing practices to children depend on appropriate intersectoral action and dialogue, sound governance and accountability mechanisms, as well as a focus on equity and a child's rights approach. These are all elements at the heart of the new health policy framework for the WHO European Region, Health 2020, which supports action across government and society for health.

I strongly believe that the trends in childhood obesity can be reversed. This report [Marketing of foods high in fat, salt and sugar to children: update 2012–2013], although a small step in providing evidence on the trends and policy processes in tackling one of the determinants of childhood obesity, illustrates the enormous progress that has been made in recent years. At the same time, it highlights how collaboration among Member States can trigger decisive action.

To be effective, the initiative to reduce the exposure of children to the marketing of foods and non-alcoholic beverages should be part of a broader package that needs to include: scaling up and adopting the WHO Childhood Obesity Surveillance Initiative; introducing appropriate governance mechanisms with an intersectoral perspective to streamline action and implement a best buys approach to tackling childhood obesity; and ensuring that childhood obesity strategies and non-communicable disease policies are connected and interact appropriately with strategies to reduce inequality.

Zsuzsanna Jakab

WHO Regional Director for Europe

Source: Marketing of foods high in fat, salt and sugar to children: update 2012–2013, http://www.euro.who.int/en/what-we-publish/ abstracts/ marketing-of-foods-high-in-fat,-salt-and-sugar-to-children-update-20122013

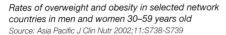

	Men	Women
Brazil		
Urban	49%	45%
Rural	25%	43%
India		
Urban		19.9%
Bangladesh		
Urban	5.4%	5.4%
Rural	3.7%	3.6%
Russia	30.3%	50.3%
USA	61%*	

*Rates of overweight and obesity in selected network
countries in men and women 30–59 years old*
Source: Asia Pacific J Clin Nutr 2002;11:S738-S739

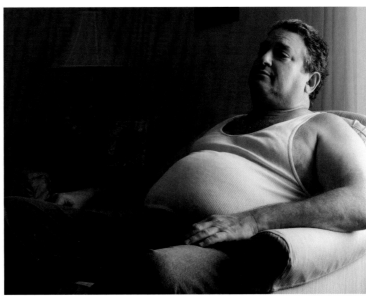

The world is getting wider

It is lunchtime at Eastside Elementary School in Clinton, Mississippi, the fattest state in the fattest country in the Western world. Uniformed lunch ladies stand at the ready. Nine-year-olds line up dutifully, trays in hand. Yes to chocolate milk, yes to breaded chicken sandwiches, yes to baked beans, yes to orange jelly, no to salad. Bowls of iceberg lettuce and tomatoes sit rim to rim, rejected. Regina Ducksworth, in charge of Clinton's lunch menu, sighs. "Broccoli is very popular," she says, reassuringly. Persuading children to eat vegetables is hardly a new struggle, nor would it seem to rank high on the list of global priorities. In an age of plenty, individuals have the luxury of eating what they like. Yet America, for all its libertarian ethos, is now worrying about how its citizens eat and how much exercise they take. It has become an issue of national concern.

Two thirds of American adults are overweight. This is defined as having a body mass index (BMI, a common measure of obesity) of 25 or more, which for a man standing 175 cm (5 feet 9 inches) tall means a weight of 77 kg (170 pounds) or more. Alarmingly, 36% of adults and 17% of children are not just overweight but obese, with a BMI of at least 30, meaning they weigh 92 kg or more at the same height. If current trends continue, by 2030 nearly half of American adults could be obese.

Americans may be shocked by these numbers, but for the rest of the world they fit a stereotype. Hamburgers, sodas and sundaes are considered as American as the Stars and Stripes. Food at state fairs is American cuisine at its most exuberantly sickening. At the Mississippi fair, a deep-fried Oreo biscuit's crispy exterior gives way to soft dough, sweet cream and chocolate goo. It is irresistible.

The rest of the world should not scoff at Americans, because belts in many other places are stretched too, as shown by new data from Majid Ezzati of Imperial College, London, and Gretchen Stevens of the World Health Organization (WHO). Some continental Europeans remain relatively slender. Swiss women are the slimmest, and most French women don't get fat, as they like to brag (though nearly 15% do). But in Britain 25% of all women are obese, with men following close behind at 24%. Czech men take the European biscuit: 30% are obese.

And it is not just the rich world that is too big for its own good. The world's two main hubs for blub are the Pacific Islands and the Gulf region. Mexican adults are as fat as their northern neighbors. In Brazil the tall and slender are being superseded by the pudgy, with 53% of adults overweight in 2008. Even in China, which has seen devastating famine within living memory, one adult in four is overweight or obese, with higher rates among city-dwellers. In all, according to Dr Ezzati, in 2008 about 1.5 billion adults, or roughly one third of the world's adult population, were overweight or obese. Obesity rates were nearly double those in 1980.

61

Fat of the land

Not long ago the world's main worry was that people had too little to eat. Malnourishment remains a serious concern in some regions: some 16% of the world's children, mainly in sub-Saharan Africa and South Asia, were underweight in 2010. But 20 years earlier the figure was 24%. In a study of 36 developing countries, based on data from 1992 to 2000, Barry Popkin of the University of North Carolina found that most of them had more overweight than underweight women.

The clearest explanation of this extraordinary modern phenomenon comes from a doctor who lived in the 5th century BCE. "As a general rule," Hippocrates wrote, "the constitutions and the habits of a people follow the nature of the land where they live." Men and women of all ages and many cultures did not choose gluttony and sloth over abstemiousness and hard work in the space of just a few decades. Rather, their surroundings changed dramatically, and with them their behavior.

Much of the shift is due to economic growth. BMI rises in line with GDP up to $5,000 per person per year, then the correlation ends. Greater wealth means that bicycles are abandoned for motorbikes and cars, and work in the fields is swapped for sitting at a desk. In rich countries the share of the population that gets insufficient exercise is more than twice as high as in poor ones.

Very importantly, argues Boyd Swinburn of Deakin University in Melbourne, diets change. Families can afford to eat more food of all kinds, and particularly those high in fat and sugar. Mothers spend more time at work and less time cooking. Food companies push their products harder. Richard Wrangham of Harvard University says that heavily processed food may have helped increase obesity rates. Softer foods take less energy to break down and finely milled grains can be digested more completely, so the body absorbs more calories.

These global changes react with local factors to create different problems in different regions. Counter-intuitively, in some countries malnutrition is leading to higher obesity rates. Undernourished mothers produce babies who are predisposed to gaining weight easily, which makes children in fast-developing countries particularly prone to getting fat.

In Mexico unreliable tap water and savvy marketing have helped make the country the world's leading guzzler of Coca-Cola: the average adult consumed 728 servings last year. In America junk-food calories are often cheaper than healthy ones. Suburban sprawl and the universal availability of food have made the car the new dining room. In the Middle East, Bedouin traditions of hosting and feasting have combined with wealth to make overeating a nightly habit. Any inclination to exercise is discouraged by heat and cultural restrictions. In Beijing teenagers and office workers cram the fast-food restaurants along Wangfujing. Even home-cooked Chinese meals contain more meat and oil than they used to. Doting grandparents shower edible treats on scarce grandchildren.

Together, these disparate changes have caused more and more people to become fat. Many cultures used to view a large girth with approval, as a sign of prosperity. But obesity has costs. It lowers workers' productivity and in the longer term raises the risk of myriad ailments, including diabetes, heart disease, strokes and some cancers; it also affects mental health. In America, obesity-related illness accounted for one fifth of total healthcare spending in 2005, according to one paper.

A new global health study, led by Christopher Murray of the University of Washington, shows that since 1990 obesity has grown faster than any other cause of disease. For women a high BMI is now the third-largest driver of illness. At the same time childhood mortality has dropped and the average age of the world's population has risen rapidly. In combination these trends may mark a shift in public-health priorities. Increasingly, early death is less of a worry than decades spent alive and sick.

It is plain that obesity has become a huge problem, that the factors influencing it are fiendishly hard to untangle and that reversing it will involve difficult choices. Radical moves such as banning junk food would infringe individuals' freedom to eat what they like. Instead, some governments are cautiously prodding their citizens to eat less and exercise more, and food companies are offering at least some healthier foods.

In a few places obesity rates seem to be leveling, but for now waistlines in most countries continue to widen unabated. Jiang He and his colleagues at Tulane University have estimated that by 2030 the global number of overweight and obese people may double to 3.3 billion. That would have huge implications for individuals, governments, employers, food companies and makers of pharmaceuticals.

Source: Charlotte Howard, Special Report: The world is getting wider, www.theeconomist.com, December 2012

Why lower-income households suffer the most

In many low-income countries, the populations affected most by the problem of obesity and NCDs are the wealthy and well-educated people that have changed their traditional dietary patterns. One reason for this shift is the increased capability that comes with rising incomes to purchase a more diverse diet, including more protein and fat, combined with changing tastes. In developed countries, however another reason for the change in diet is that poor households lack access to more nutritious foods, either because they are not readily available (cf. the section on food deserts in Chapter Three) or they cannot afford them. The more inexpensive foods tend to be high in fats and sugars, so they may be energy-dense but are typically nutrient-sparse.

It is not unusual to find households containing overweight people who are also anemic, or who have significant deficiencies in zinc, vitamin A, and other micronutrients. It can be difficult to acknowledge such dietary inadequacies, as anemia is not immediately apparent to the eye. Calorie-rich but nutrient-poor fast food is one obvious culprit, but there are other factors too. Snacking, for instance, is another major problem and it has become, in developed countries, the 'fourth full meal' of the day – a meal that is surplus to requirements.

The long road to behavior change

In the United States and Europe, much attention was given to the topic of nutrition at the end of World War II. This was partly on account of the lessons learned about the relationship between nutrition and health in the extreme conditions of wartime, and partly on account of a general concern about how to feed a rapidly growing global population during a time of general peace. In the United States, as elsewhere in the West, the people who had experienced the war wanted a better life – less work, more food, more leisure, more consumer goods. The creation and satisfaction of consumer desire became a key driver of the economy in the boom years of post-war peace and plenty. While cheap food was made readily available, however, the long-term consequences of the new fast-food culture were not understood. We now have a situation whereby the United States feeds itself too well – and at the same time not well enough. In the United States, around two thirds of adults are either overweight or obese. Non-Hispanic, African-Americans and Mexican-Americans in the US tend to have higher rates of obesity linked to low incomes. And

the rest of the world is following the American model, with alarming consequences: the UN reports a worldwide figure of $190 billion (US) worth of workdays lost and healthcare costs as a direct result of obesity and its related non-communicable diseases.

Treating people who are already obese is not easy, however. Studies show that only 5–8% of people who go on weight reduction diets keep the weight off long-term (defined as 5–10 years or more). There is a long-running study called the 'Weight Maintainers Study' in the United States which sets participants the goal of losing 50lb and keeping this weight off for five years or more. The weight maintainers have succeeded in keeping the weight off by following a combination of closely monitoring their food intake, routinely eating breakfast and having, on average, one hour of exercise per day. This specific set of behaviors is proven to work. Nevertheless, for many people, adoption of these behaviors is difficult due to money and time limitations. Thus gaining weight is easy but alas losing it is a very different matter.

Further reading

World Health Organization. Obesity: Preventing and managing the global epidemic. Report of a WHO consultation. WHO Tech Rep Ser 2000;894:1-252. Geneva: WHO, 2000.

Birch LL, Parker L, Burns A (eds). Early Childhood Obesity Prevention Policies. Washington, DC: Institute of Medicine, 2011.

63

WHO's recommendations

Overweight and obesity, as well as their related non-communicable diseases, are largely preventable. Supportive environments and communities are fundamental in shaping people's choices, making healthier foods and regular physical activity the easiest choice (accessible, available and affordable), and therefore preventing obesity.

At the individual level, people can: limit energy intake from total fats and sugars; increase consumption of fruit and vegetables, as well as legumes, whole grains and nuts; engage in regular physical activity (60 minutes a day for children and 150 minutes per week for adults).

Individual responsibility can only have its full effect where people have access to a healthy lifestyle. Therefore, at the societal level it is important to: support individuals in following the recommendations above, through sustained political commitment and the collaboration of many public and private stakeholders; make regular physical activity and healthier dietary choices available, affordable and easily accessible to all - especially the poorest individuals.

The food industry can play a significant role in promoting healthy diets by: reducing the fat, sugar and salt content of processed foods; ensuring that healthy and nutritious choices are available and affordable to all consumers; practicing responsible marketing especially those aimed at children and teenagers; ensuring the availability of healthy food choices and supporting regular physical activity practice in the workplace.

The WHO Global Strategy on Diet, Physical Activity and Health

Adopted by the World Health Assembly in 2004, the WHO Global Strategy on Diet, Physical Activity and Health describes the actions needed to support healthy diets and regular physical activity. The Strategy calls upon all stakeholders to take action at global, regional and local levels to improve diets and physical activity patterns at the population level.

WHO has developed the 2008–2013 Action Plan for the Global Strategy for the Prevention and Control of Noncommunicable Diseases to help the millions who are already affected cope with these lifelong illnesses and prevent secondary complications. This action plan aims to build on the WHO Framework Convention on Tobacco Control and the WHO Global Strategy on Diet, Physical Activity and Health. The action plan provides a roadmap to establish and strengthen initiatives for the surveillance, prevention and management of NCDs.

The Political Declaration of the High Level Meeting of the United Nations General Assembly on the Prevention and Control of Non-communicable Diseases of September 2011 recognizes the critical importance of reducing the level of exposure of individuals and populations to unhealthy diet and physical inactivity.

Source: WHO Fact Sheet 311, March 2013

My personal view

Eileen Kennedy
Professor of Nutrition, Former Dean of the Friedman School of Nutrition Science and Policy, Tufts University, Boston, USA

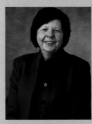

Globally we are facing an obesity epidemic of alarming proportions. Diet-related chronic diseases now account for more deaths than undernutrition. This is seen in some of the poorest countries of the world. In the past few decades traditional grain-based diets have been replaced by diets higher in total fats, saturated fats and sugars. The changing consumption patterns are occurring simultaneously with lifestyles that include less physical activity. Yet, despite the magnitude of the problem, the message has not reached policy-makers in many low-income countries. The challenge is daunting. The international community must aggressively implement multi-pronged strategies to combat overweight and obesity, while at the same time tackling undernutrition.

Chapter Five

The Economic Cost of Malnutrition

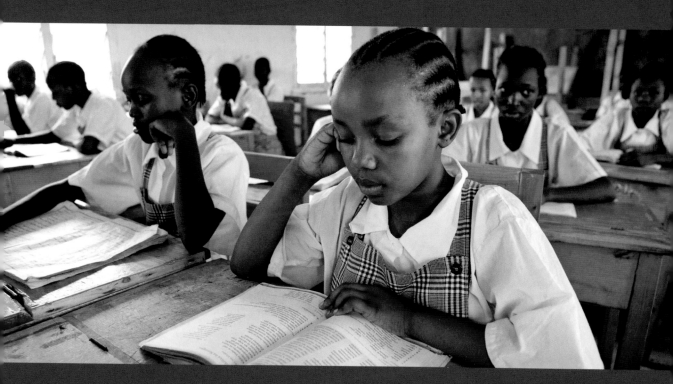

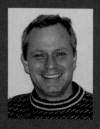

John Hoddinott

Deputy Director,
Poverty Health and Nutrition Division, International Food Policy Research Institute
(IFPRI) Washington DC, USA

"Money is a needful and precious thing, and when well used, a noble thing, but I never want you to think it is the first or only prize to strive for."

Louisa May Alcott, *American novelist (1832–1888)*

Key messages

- Chronic undernutrition and micronutrient deficiencies are prevalent across the developing world.

- In addition to its substantial human costs, undernutrition has lifelong economic consequences.

- There exist feasible solutions to many dimensions of undernutrition.

- Fighting undernutrition has considerable economic benefits, most notably in terms of improving schooling, cognitive skills and economic productivity.

- Spending that reduces both chronic undernutrition and micronutrient deficiencies is an excellent investment in economic terms; it is one of the smartest ways to spend global aid dollars.

The problem of widespread undernutrition

Around 165 million preschoolchildren suffer from chronic undernutrition. Because of inadequate food intake, repeated infection or both they fail to grow at the same rate as healthy, well-fed children. Millions more suffer from deficiencies in micronutrients such as vitamin A, iron, iodine and zinc – a phenomenon sometimes called 'hidden hunger'. Deprivation in a world of plenty is reason enough for investments that reduce undernutrition. Attacking these problems is also good economics.

Hunger, food insecurity and undernutrition

Hunger, food insecurity and undernutrition are related but not synonymous. Hunger is "A condition, in which people lack the basic food intake to provide them with the energy and nutrients for fully productive lives" (Hunger Task Force, 2003). Food security exists when all people, at all times, have physical, social and economic access to sufficient, safe and nutritious food which meets their dietary needs and food preferences for an active and healthy life (United Nations, Food and Agriculture Organization). As discussed here and elsewhere in this book, nutrients provided by food combine with other factors, including the

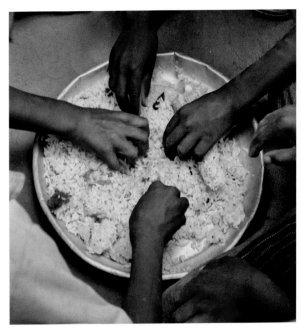

Malnourished children eating rice in Kakuma Refugee Camp, Kenya
Source: Mike Bloem Photography

health state of the person consuming the food, to produce "nutritional status." Undernutrition reflects an absence of macro- or micronutrients which may be exacerbated by debilitating health stresses such as parasites.

A powerful investment to reduce hunger and food insecurity is increased spending on agricultural research and development. This includes research that enhances drought, heat and salt tolerance, identifying and disseminating varieties with enhanced yield potential, increasing milk yields and soil diagnostics that would permit optimal combinations of organic and inorganic fertilizers. This investment has five benefit streams: i) increases in welfare gains resulting from lower prices faced by consumers; ii) welfare gains from reduced yield volatility; iii) the option value of reduced yield volatility resulting from climate change; iv) productivity gains derived from the impact of increased caloric consumption on worker productivity; and v) the income gains in adulthood resulting from reduced undernutrition in early life. An additional $8 billion dollars per year would, by 2050, reduce the number of hungry people in the world by 210 million.

Undernutrition and its consequences – physical and neurological

The first thousand days, in utero and the first two years after birth, are critical for a child's physical and neurological development. During this period, children's nutritional status is affected by the quantity and quality of food they consume. Exclusive breastfeeding in the first six months conveys critical benefits and it is vitally important that complementary foods introduced after this contain the right quantities of macronutrients – calories and protein – as well as micronutrients.

What happens when these are lacking? As discussed elsewhere in this book, children need energy to grow. Where this energy is absent, or where a child is repeatedly ill with infections that divert energy from growth while suppressing appetite, children fail to grow at a healthy rate. Studies that have followed children from infancy through to adulthood find that this lost growth is never fully regained and so these individuals end up shorter in height than they would have been if their diets had been adequate and they had not been subject to repeat infection. Vitamin A deficiencies kill. Current estimates suggest that more than 145,000 deaths in children under five occur each year because children lack vitamin A. This number has significantly declined in recent years due to the improved reach of vitamin A capsule distribution programs. Zinc deficiency affects children's physical growth and leads to increased susceptibility to a number of infections including diarrhea and pneumonia.

Both macro- and micronutrient deficiencies have insidious effects on neurological development. Iodine deficiency adversely affects development of the central nervous system leading to loss of IQ and mental retardation. Iron is needed to make brain chemicals (neurotransmitters) that aid in concentration; iron deficiency constrains cognitive development in children. Chronic undernutrition has neurological consequences that lead to cognitive impairments. The prefrontal cortex is especially vulnerable to undernutrition with the result that undernourished children can suffer from attention deficits and reduced working memory. Other neurological insults resulting from chronic undernutrition include damage to the parts of the brain responsible for spatial navigation and motor skills, The parts of the brain (axons) responsible for transmitting signals from one neuron (brain cell) to another are damaged by chronic undernutrition with the result that these signals are passed more slowly and inefficiently.

These malign effects can be exacerbated by the interactions that occur, or do not occur, between children and their caregivers. For example, delayed development of motor skills such as crawling and walking, together with lethargy and increased incidence of illness in undernourished infants, reduces their interactions with adults and with their environment.

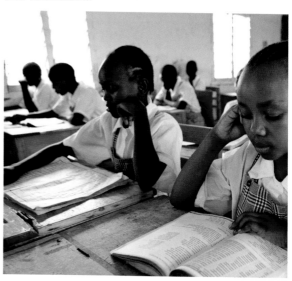

Girls in a classroom in Kakuma Refugee Camp, Kenya
Source: Mike Bloem Photography

Undernutrition and its consequences – economic

The persistently malign effects of undernutrition in early life have significant economic consequences in adulthood. A number of studies show that shorter individuals have lower earnings in adulthood although the precise reason for this – the direct effect of height on physical productivity; the social benefits associated with height – vary from place to place. There is evidence that undernutrition in early life, manifested as low birth weight, increases susceptibility to coronary heart disease, non-insulin dependent diabetes, and high blood pressure – the Barker hypothesis. However, the biggest economic consequences are those resulting from neurological damage. Studies that have followed undernourished preschoolchildren find that they attain fewer grades of schooling and develop poorer cognitive skills such as those relating to problem solving. By contrast, there is strong evidence that interventions that combat undernutrition in early life convey lifelong benefits.

Everywhere in the world, schooling and cognitive skills are vital for success in the labor market. A useful rule of thumb is that every additional grade of schooling raises wages by eight to 12 percent. So individuals without such skills and with less schooling earn lower wages, which makes it more likely that they will be poor.

The fetal programming concept

"A consequence that is also emerging more clearly is the impact of stunting and subsequent disproportionate and rapid weight gain on health later in life. These long-term effects are referred to as the fetal programming concept: Poor fetal growth, small size at birth and continued poor growth in early life followed by rapid weight gain later in childhood raises the risk of coronary heart disease, stroke, hypertension and type 2 diabetes. Attaining optimal growth before 24 months of age is desirable; becoming stunted but then gaining weight disproportionately after 24 months is likely to increase the risk of becoming overweight and developing other health problems.

"As stunted children enter adulthood with a greater propensity for developing obesity and other chronic diseases, the possibility of a burgeoning epidemic of poor health opens up, especially in transitional countries experiencing increasing urbanization and shifts in diet and lifestyle. This epidemiological transition could create new economic and social challenges in many low- and middle-income countries where stunting is prevalent, especially among poorer population groups."

Source: UNICEF Improving Child Nutrition 2013

Case study

A series of studies led by Professor Reynaldo Martorell at Emory University, have shed light on the long-term benefits of improving nutritional status in young children.

More than four decades ago, between 1969 and 1977, two nutritional supplements - a high-protein-energy drink called *Atole* and a low-energy drink devoid of protein called *Fresco* – were provided to preschoolchildren in four villages in eastern Guatemala. Between 2002 and 2004, individuals who had been exposed to this intervention were traced throughout Guatemala and interviewed about their schooling, marital histories, living conditions and participation in the labor market. They took reading, vocabulary and problem-solving tests. Their heights and weights were measured as were the heights and weights of their children. Because these supplements were randomly assigned across villages, and because of the care with which the intervention was implemented and the wealth

of additional information that was collected, it is possible to draw causal inferences of the effect of the high-protein-energy drink.

For both men and women, access to *atole* significantly raised scores on reading, vocabulary tests and on tests of problem-solving ability more than twenty-five years after the intervention had concluded. For men, access to *atole* increased wages by more than 40 percent. (There was no impact on women's wages largely because relatively few women participated in work outside the home.) The benefits of *atole* were intergenerational. Offspring of women exposed to *atole* had higher birth weights and were taller compared with offspring of women exposed to *fresco*.

The Guatemala study provides powerful evidence of the long-term investments that reduce chronic undernutrition.

The economics of reducing undernutrition

The human and economic costs of undernutrition would seem to make a compelling case for investments – purposive actions by governments, non-governmental organizations and the private sector – to reduce undernutrition. Some of these investments – such as increasing girls' schooling, improving the health and status of women ("healthy mothers for healthy children") and improved water and sanitation – are important development objectives in their own right. But what about direct interventions to reduce macro- and micronutrient deficiencies? Are these good investments?

A number of studies have looked at the costs of these investments relative to the economic benefits that they would provide. There is an element of uncertainty surrounding these calculations – as there is with any benefit: cost analysis – because they rely on estimating the costs of these interventions today and calculating the stream of economic benefits that accrue over the decades that follow.

With that caution in mind, a good economic investment is an investment where the benefit:cost ratio exceeds one; that is to say that for every dollar spent today on investments to reduce undernutrition, the future stream of economic benefits valued in today's terms exceeds one dollar. Measured in this way, there is overwhelming evidence that investments to reduce micronutrient deficiencies and chronic undernutrition have high benefit:cost ratios:

- Every dollar spent iodizing salt generates $30 in economic benefits;

- Every dollar spent on iron supplements for mothers and children aged six to 24 months generates $24 in economic benefits

- Every dollar spent on vitamin A generates economic benefits estimated to be $40 or more

- Reducing chronic undernutrition requires bundling micronutrient interventions such as those that reduce vitamin A, iodine and iron deficiencies with the provision of other micronutrients (such as zinc powders needed to reduce the duration and severity of diarrhea), and energy-dense foods. Also important is communication with mothers and other caregivers about the importance of these for healthy child growth. The costs associated with doing so vary across countries as do the benefits but in a typical developing country, every dollar spent on this bundle generates around $18 in economic benefits

By the standards of economics, these are impressively high benefit:cost ratios. Not only that, the costs of these investments are trivially low. In addition to current expenditures spent combatting undernutrition, an additional annual investment of about $650 million dollars a year – less than two dollars from every North American and western European – would be enough to eliminate vitamin A deficiency in the 95 million preschoolchildren who are vitamin A deficient, iodine deficiencies affecting nearly two billion people and anemia affecting 80 million pregnant women. A larger investment is needed for the bundle of interventions needed to reduce chronic undernutrition – current estimates suggest that around nine and half billion dollars per year would reach 90% of children in the 34 countries that account for 90% of the burden of undernutrition in the developing world.

The Copenhagen Consensus

The origin of the Copenhagen Consensus dates back to 2002, and a small team of people headed by Bjorn Lomborg, then Director of the Danish Environmental Assessment Institute. Funded for a period of time by the Danish government, the Copenhagen Consensus Centre is a think tank which "commissions and conducts new research and analysis into competing spending priorities. In particular we focus on the international community's effort to solve the world's biggest challenges and on how to do this in the most cost-efficient manner."

In 2004, 2008 and 2012, the Copenhagen Consensus Centre held a series of global conferences. At each, an expert panel, including four Nobel Laureates, looked at twelve major global challenges, deliberating the question: "If you had $75 billion for worthwhile causes, where should you start?" The experts were informed by 30 economic research papers by eminent scholars which provided cost-benefit analyses for a range of potential interventions. In each round, the panel found investments to reduce micronutrient deficiencies and chronic hunger to be among the best investments that could be made with these funds. In 2012 the panel ranked 'Interventions to Reduce Chronic Undernutrition in Preschoolers' to be the highest-ranking solution.

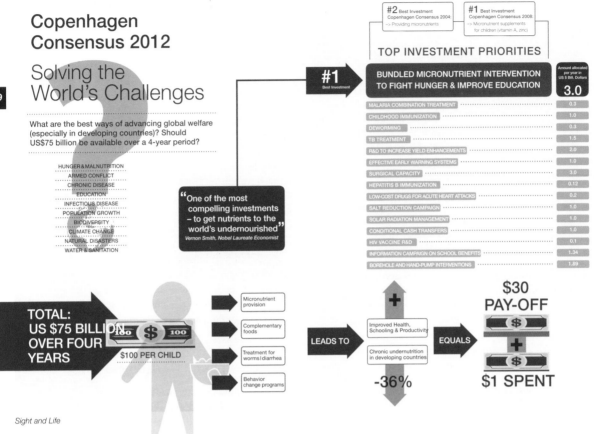

Copenhagen Consensus 2012

Solving the World's Challenges

What are the best ways of advancing global welfare (especially in developing countries)? Should US$75 billion be available over a 4-year period?

HUNGER & MALNUTRITION
ARMED CONFLICT
CHRONIC DISEASE
EDUCATION
INFECTIOUS DISEASE
POPULATION GROWTH
BIODIVERSITY
CLIMATE CHANGE
NATURAL DISASTERS
WATER & SANITATION

"One of the most compelling investments – to get nutrients to the world's undernourished"
Vernon Smith, Nobel Laureate Economist

#2 Best Investment
Copenhagen Consensus 2004:
-> Providing micronutrients

#1 Best Investment
Copenhagen Consensus 2008:
-> Micronutrient supplements for children (vitamin A, zinc)

TOP INVESTMENT PRIORITIES

	Amount allocated per year in US $ Bill. Dollars
#1 Best Investment — BUNDLED MICRONUTRIENT INTERVENTION TO FIGHT HUNGER & IMPROVE EDUCATION	3.0
MALARIA COMBINATION TREATMENT	0.3
CHILDHOOD IMMUNIZATION	1.0
DEWORMING	0.3
TB TREATMENT	1.5
R&D TO INCREASE YIELD ENHANCEMENTS	2.0
EFFECTIVE EARLY WARNING SYSTEMS	1.0
SURGICAL CAPACITY	3.0
HEPATITIS B IMMUNIZATION	0.12
LOW-COST DRUGS FOR ACUTE HEART ATTACKS	0.2
SALT REDUCTION CAMPAIGN	1.0
SOLAR RADIATION MANAGEMENT	1.0
CONDITIONAL CASH TRANSFERS	1.0
HIV VACCINE R&D	0.1
INFORMATION CAMPAIGN ON SCHOOL BENEFITS	1.34
BOREHOLE AND HAND-PUMP INTERVENTIONS	1.89

TOTAL: US $75 BILLION OVER FOUR YEARS

$100 PER CHILD

Micronutrient provision
Complementary foods
Treatment for worms | diarrhea
Behavior change programs

LEADS TO

Improved Health, Schooling & Productivity +

Chronic undernutrition in developing countries –36%

EQUALS

$30 PAY-OFF
+
$1 SPENT

Sight and Life

The Developmental Course of Human Brain Development

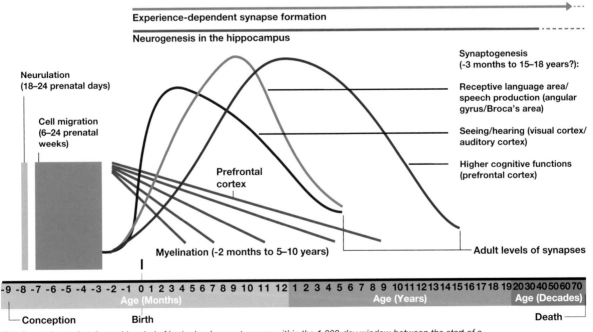

Experience-dependent synapse formation

Neurogenesis in the hippocampus

Neurulation (18–24 prenatal days)

Cell migration (6–24 prenatal weeks)

Prefrontal cortex

Myelination (-2 months to 5–10 years)

Synaptogenesis (-3 months to 15–18 years?):

Receptive language area/ speech production (angular gyrus/Broca's area)

Seeing/hearing (visual cortex/ auditory cortex)

Higher cognitive functions (prefrontal cortex)

Adult levels of synapses

-9 -8 -7 -6 -5 -4 -3 -2 -1 0 1 2 3 4 5 6 7 8 9 10 11 12 | 1 2 3 4 5 6 7 8 9 10 11 12 13 14 15 16 17 18 19 20 30 40 50 60 70

Age (Months)   Age (Years)   Age (Decades)

Conception   Birth   Death

This figure shows that the rapid period of brain development occurs within the 1,000-day window between the start of a woman's pregnancy and her child's second birthday.

Thomson, Nelson (2001) Developmental Science and the Media

Global estimates of undernourishment (hunger) 1969-2010

Period	Number of undernourished (millions)	Prevalence (percentage)
1969-71	875	33
1979-81	850	25
1990-92	848	16
1995-97	792	14
2000-02	836	14
2006-08	850	13
2009	1023*	18
2010	925*	16

FAO, State of Food Insecurity in the World, 2012

Regional estimates of undernourishment 1990-2008

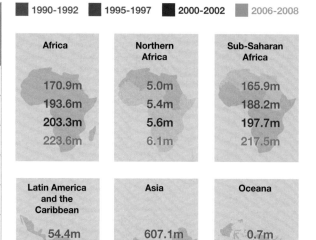

■ 1990-1992   ■ 1995-1997   ■ 2000-2002   ■ 2006-2008

Africa
170.9m
193.6m
203.3m
223.6m

Northern Africa
5.0m
5.4m
5.6m
6.1m

Sub-Saharan Africa
165.9m
188.2m
197.7m
217.5m

Latin America and the Caribbean
54.4m
53.4m
50.8m
47.0m

Asia
607.1m
526.2m
565.7m
567.8m

Oceana
0.7m
0.8m
1.0m
1.0m

Hunger and Malnutrition, Copenhagen Consensus 2012

Projected change in World Commodity Prices presented as a percent change between baseline 2010 and baseline 2050

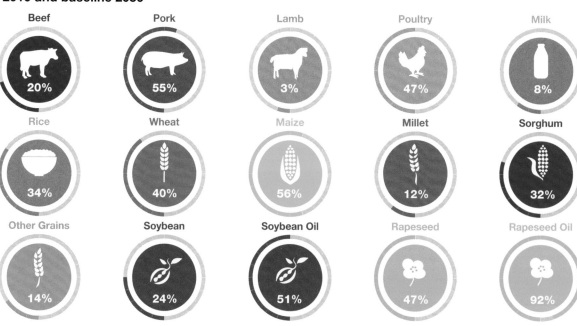

Beef 20% Pork 55% Lamb 3% Poultry 47% Milk 8%

Rice 34% Wheat 40% Maize 56% Millet 12% Sorghum 32%

Other Grains 14% Soybean 24% Soybean Oil 51% Rapeseed 47% Rapeseed Oil 92%

Hunder and Malnutrition, Copenhagen Consensus 2012

Per child cost of interventions to reduce stunting and mortality at age 36 months

Intervention	Child age range (months)	Cost per unit	Total cost per child
Community based nutrition programs that provide information on breastfeeding, complementary feeding, handwashing, and distribute micronutrient powders and iron-folate supplements	0–59	$7.50 per child	$7.50
Vitamin A supplementation	6-59	$1.20 per year	$4.80
Therapeutic zinc supplementation for management of diarrhea	6-59	$1.00 per year (assumes two or three treatments per year)	$4.00
Multiple micronutrient powders	6-23	$3.60 per course; 3 courses recommended	$10.80
Deworming	12-59	$0.25 per round; one round recommended per year	$1.00
Iron-folic acid supplementation for mothers during pregnancy		$2.00 per pregnancy	$2.00
Iron fortification of staples	12-59	$0.20 per year	$0.80
Universal salt iodization	12-59	$0.05 per year	$0.20
Providing complementary foods to 80 percent of children in South Asia, 50 percent in Africa and East Asia, 10 percent elsewhere	6-23	$0.11 per day $0.14 per day in India	$56.88
Community based management of severe acute malnutrition	6-59		$8.13

Hunger and Malnutrition, Copenhagen Consensus 2012

Benefit: cost estimages of investments that reduce stunting

	Discount rate	23.8% income increase		15% income increase	
		5%	3%	5%	3%
Bangladesh	Increased income, NPV:	3647	7165	2303	4523
	Cost:	96.1	96.1	96.1	96.1
	Benefit: Cost ratio:	**38.0**	**74.6**	**24.0**	**47.1**
Ethiopia	Increased income, NPV:	2289	4496	1445	2838
	Cost:	96.1	96.1	96.1	96.1
	Benefit: Cost ratio:	**23.8**	**46.8**	**15.0**	**29.5**
Kenya	Increased income, NPV:	3713	7295	2344	4605
	Cost:	96.1	96.1	96.1	96.1
	Benefit: Cost ratio:	**38.6**	**75.9**	**24.4**	**47.9**
India	Increased income, NPV:	7875	15470	4972	9767
	Cost:	111.62	111.62	111.62	111.62
	Benefit: Cost ratio:	**70.6**	**138.6**	**44.5**	**87.5**

Hunger and Malnutrition, Copenhagen Consensus 2012

NPV = net present value

Baseline projections for people at risk of hunger in 2010, 2025 and 2050

Region	People at Risk of Hunger (millions)		
Projected Year	2010	2025	2050
East Asia and Pacific	177	131	122
Europe and Central Asia	23	23	21
Latin America and the Caribbean	60	61	45
Middle East and North Africa	17	21	24
South Asia	318	310	235
Sub-Saharan Africa	240	275	268
Developing	835	821	716
Developed	49	50	50
World	884	870	766

Hunger and Malnutrition, Copenhagen Consensus 2012

Baseline projections of malnourished children in 2010, 2025 and 2050

Region	Number of Malnourished Children (millions)		
Projected Year	2010	2025	2050
East Asia and Pacific	20	13	8
Europe and Central Asia	4	3	3
Latin America and the Caribbean	8	7	4
Middle East and North Africa	4	3	2
South Asia	74	65	50
Sub-Saharan Africa	41	44	39
Developing	150	135	106
Developed	12	12	12
World	163	147	118

Hunger and Malnutrition, Copenhagen Consensus 2012

Benefit: cost ratios of micronutrient interventions

26 Fe Iron — Intervention: Supplements, mothers and children 6-24 months

Previous Estimates	New Estimates	Current Estimates of cost per beneficiary
-	23.8 RAJ	$0.96 RAJ

26 Fe Iron — Intervention: Supplements, pregnant mothers

Previous Estimates	New Estimates	Current Estimates of cost per beneficiary
82-140 RAJ	8.1 HOR	
-		$2.00 HOR 2010

26 Fe Iron — Intervention: Fortification, general

Previous Estimates	New Estimates	Current Estimates of cost per beneficiary
7.8 HAR	-	-

26 Fe Iron — Intervention: Fortification of wheat flour

Previous Estimates	New Estimates	Current Estimates of cost per beneficiary
	9.1 HOR	
-	6.7 CASEY 2011	$0.17 HOR

26 Fe Iron — Intervention: Home fortification

Previous Estimates	New Estimates	Current Estimates of cost per beneficiary
-	37 HOR	$1.20 HOR

26 Fe Iron — Intervention: Biofortification

Previous Estimates	New Estimates	Current Estimates of cost per beneficiary
11.6-19 BAH		
16.7 HAR	-	<$0.01 HOR

53 I Iodine — Intervention: Salt Iodization

Previous Estimates	New Estimates	Current Estimates of cost per beneficiary
15-520 BAH		
30 HAR	81 RAJ	$0.05 HAR

53 26 I Fe Iodine & Iron — Intervention: Doubly fortified salt

Previous Estimates	New Estimates	Current Estimates of cost per beneficiary
	2.5 RAJ	
-	2-5 HOR	$0.25 HOR

A Vitamin A — Intervention: Supplement

Previous Estimates	New Estimates	Current Estimates of cost per beneficiary
4.3-43 BAH		
6.1-250 HAR	12.5 RAJ	$0.29 RAJ

30 Zn Zinc — Intervention: Supplement

Previous Estimates	New Estimates	Current Estimates of cost per beneficiary
-	2.85 RAJ	$1.26 RAJ

Hunger and Malnutrition, Copenhagen Consensus 2012. **Casey** *GJ, Sartori D, Horton SE, Phuc TQ, Phu LB, et al, 2011. Weekly Iron-Folic Acid supplementation with Regular Deworming Is Cost-Effective in Preventing Anaemia in Women of Reproductive Age in Vietnam. PLoS ONE 6(9) 23723. doi:10.1371/journal.pone.0023723.* **BAH** *Behrman, J., Alderman, H., and Hoddinott, J., 2004. Hunger and Malnutrition, in B. Lomborg (ed.) Global crises, Global solutions, Cambridge University Press, Cambridge UK.* **HAR** *Horton, S., H. Alderman and J. Rivera, 2008. Hunger and Malnutrition. Copenhagen Consensus 2008 Challenge Paper, Copenhagen Consensus Center, Copenhagen.* **HOR** *Horton, S., A. Wesley and M.G. Venkatesh Mannar, 2011. Double-fortified salt reduces anemia, benefit: cost ratio is modestly favorable. Food Policy, 36(5): 581-587.* **HOR** *2010 Horton, S., M. Shekar, C. McDonald, A. Mahal and J. Brooks, 2010. Scaling up nutrition: What will it cost? World Bank, Washington DC.* **RAJ** *Rajkumar, A.S., C. Gaukler, and J. Tilahun, 2012. Combating Malnutrition in Ethiopia: An Evidence-Based Approach for Sustained Results World Bank: Washington DC.*

73

Malnutrition and obesity

The word "malnutrition" encompasses undernutrition, deficiencies in macro- and micronutrients, and what is somewhat inelegantly termed overnutrition, excessive caloric intake, exacerbated by diseases such as diabetes and low levels of physical activity. Overweight and obese individuals are one manifestation of overnutrition. Overweight and obesity are significant public health problems in much of the developed world and increasingly in middle income countries such as Brazil and Mexico. Across the developing world, however, undernutrition is the major form of malnutrition.

An astonishing return on investment

"Improving nutrition is in fact a precondition to achieving many of the Millennium Development Goals (MDGs): eradicating poverty and hunger, reducing child mortality, improving maternal health, combating disease, empowering women and achieving universal primary education.

"Research shows that children who are well nourished, especially in the critical 1,000 day window between conception and the child's second birthday, receive the strong start in life they need to grow, fight disease, learn more in school, and earn more as adults. They also grow up to help lift their countries out of poverty: a 2010 study found that investing in nutrition can increase a country's GDP by at least 2–3 percent each year. And in May of this year, the Copenhagen Consensus panel of experts, which included no fewer than four Nobel Laureates, found that providing micronutrients to children under five is the single smartest way to spend global aid dollars. Every $1 spent yields $30 – an astonishing return on investment ratio by any measure. We cannot improve health and promote development without addressing micronutrient deficiencies. Micronutrients have a key role to play in nourishing the world's people, building strong families and creating vibrant and economically sustainable communities."

Klaus Kraemer, Sight and Life

My personal view

John Hoddinott
Deputy Director,
Poverty Health and Nutrition Division, International Food Policy Research Institute (IFPRI) Washington DC, USA

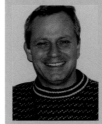

There is intrinsic value in eliminating undernutrition – it is simply the right thing to do. But beyond this, it is good economics too. Investments in reducing chronic undernutrition and micronutrient deficiencies have considerable economic benefits.

Further reading

Behrman J, Alderman H, Hoddinott J. Hunger and malnutrition. In: Lomborg B (ed) Global crisis, global solutions. Cambridge: Cambridge University Press, 2004.

Horton S, Shekar M, McDonald C et al. Scaling up nutrition: What will it cost? Washington, DC: World Bank, 2010.

Hoddinott J, Rosegrant M, Torero M. Investments to reduce hunger and undernutrition. In: Lomborg B (ed) Copenhagen Consensus 2012. Cambridge: Cambridge University Press, 2013.

Hoddinott J, Maluccio J, Behrman J et al. Effect of a nutrition intervention during early childhood on economic productivity in Guatemalan adults. Lancet 2008;371:411-416.

Chapter Six

Best Practice in Nutrition

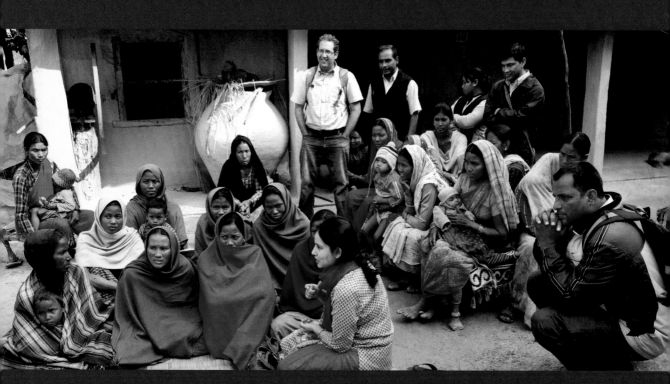

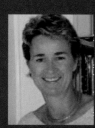

Victoria Quinn

Senior Vice President of Programs, Helen Keller International, New York, USA

Adjunct Associate Professor, Friedman School of Nutrition Science and Policy, Boston, USA

Key messages

- Undernutrition is a complex and multifaceted phenomenon, and is not limited to the developing world.

- Undernutrition does not have a single cause, nor does it have a single solution.

- The Conceptual Framework of Young Child Nutrition provides a clear and coherent way of understanding the causes of undernutrition and where we might intervene, though to do so requires that we carefully assess and analyze the local situation to inform any actions that might be taken.

- At the national level, increased government investment in proven nutrition-specific and nutrition-sensitive interventions is essential for improving nutrition.

- At the family level, women have a critical role to play in improving nutrition.

The focus of this chapter is on child undernutrition, which is manifested as growth deficits in children (stunted height or underweight) or in clinical deficiencies in micronutrients (e.g., vitamin A deficiency, iron deficiencies). Although not discussed in detail in this chapter, with changing dietary practices due to a variety of reasons, childhood overweight in developing regions is becoming an increasingly important contributor to adult obesity, diabetes, and non-communicable diseases.[1]

When children do not grow adequately due to undernutrition they suffer from deficits in linear growth and become too short for their age, or in other words "stunted". Stunting is defined as a height-for-age ratio that is more than two standard deviations below the international standards produced by the World Health Organization. Once a child becomes stunted due to sub-optimal nutrition during pregnancy and the first two years of life, there is little opportunity for catch-up growth later on. Literature now exists on the immense negative consequences of stunting, which range from increased under-five mortality through reduced IQ, poor school performance, and reduced worker productivity later in life, to increased risk of adult non-communicable diseases.[2]

Evidence also exists today that shows the most critical time to intervene to prevent undernutrition and stunting is during the *first thousand days* from conception until a child's second birthday. During pregnancy, poor maternal nutrition leads to low birth weight babies who are at higher risk of stunting. Providing women with support for optimal nutrition even before they become pregnant when they are adolescents girls, and continuing this support through gestation and after the baby is born – including optimal infant and young child feeding until his/her second birthday – is critical to promote good nutrition and healthy growth.

Confusion before enlightenment: a short history of dealing with undernutrition

For decades, there have been many different schools of thought as to the nature, causes and consequences of undernutrition in developing regions of the world, which in turn led to changing views as to what should be done about it. As one nutrition expert put it: *"New paradigms in public health nutrition have repeatedly replaced one other [sic] in the second half of the 20th century. This convulsive process continues"*.[3]

The discovery of vitamins and minerals in the early part of the 1900s focused interest on the micronutrient aspects of what was believed to constitute a healthy diet, with the absence of these thought to lead to poor health. During pre-war British colonial times, the causes of undernutrition in the people of the colonies fluctuated from being viewed as either poverty (putting the colonial powers at blame) or ignorance (putting mothers themselves at blame).[4] In Gold Coast (pre-independent Ghana), the British medical doctor Dr Cecily Williams discovered kwashiorkor, which she believed was the result of a protein deficiency in a child's die. Kwashiorkor was later proclaimed to be the most serious and widespread nutritional disorder in children known to medical or nutritional science. Therefore for many years, particularly from 1950 to the mid-70s, much of global nutrition attention in developing regions was based on the belief that protein deficiency was the cause of poor nutrition. Much effort and many resources were placed on increasing the production and consumption of protein. This obsession with protein deficiency was later de-bunked by Professor Donald McLaren in his famous 1972 Lancet article where he referred to this as the 'great protein fiasco': *"The concept of the much-publicized world protein "gap", "crisis", or "problem" arose from the description of kwashiorkor in Africa in the 1930s and the assumption, which has turned out to be wrong, that malnutrition in children takes this form throughout the world. As a result, measures to detect protein deficiency and treat and prevent it by dietary means have been pursued until the present time. The price that has had to be paid for these mistakes is only beginning to be realized."*[5]

In later years, following the establishment of the United Nations, more emphasis was placed on the structural causes of poor nutrition, culminating in the noble but naïve declaration of the 1974 World Food Conference that hunger and malnutrition would be eliminated within one decade (World Food Conference 1974, resolution V). An era of multi-sectoral nutrition planning followed from this time up through the early 1980s, with lively and often contentious debate ensuing among international nutrition experts on how successful, or not, these attempts were.[6] As it transpired, the multi-sectoral nutrition plans produced were extremely complicated and impossible to implement. Nor did they factor in political determinants, including whether political will from government leadership or planners in non-health sectors existed or whether resources were available and would be committed to fund the lofty recommendations made.[4]

By the mid-1980s, interest in community-based nutrition planning was gaining momentum. This continued for about a decade, with some useful lessons learned from UNICEF's work with the Government of Tanzania in the Iringa region of that country.[7] From the mid-1990s, the focus on nutrition in developing regions dramatically shifted to hidden hunger and micronutrient deficiencies.[3] Soon thereafter, global efforts, including resources, aligned to reach vulnerable populations with micronutrient supplementation.

In summary, the nutrition community has shifted its position over the decades for a variety of reasons including evolving scientific knowledge, accumulating field experience on what has worked, and differing ethical positions.[3] One undercurrent that has existed through the decades has been the existence of two schools of thought – one that viewed poor nutrition as a structural issue related to poverty, and the other that viewed it as a technical issue, for example, resulting from a specific deficiency that could be addressed with a health-oriented action (e.g. a pill).[4] Another observation is that over time, professionals from the health sector (e.g. nutritionists and medical doctors) and food scientists have dominated the dialogue. In other words, there has been a relative absence of voices from other disciplines important for nutrition, particularly agriculturalists and economists, whose actions could have a massive impact on not just food availability but also the economic access of families to adequate food (in terms of both quality and quantity) through their own production, purchases or trade.

Coming to consensus

By the late 1980s and early 1990s, a consensus began to form on the nature of child undernutrition. This consensus was informed by the field experiences of UNICEF and the Government of Tanzania in Iringa, who implemented a large-scale community nutrition program, and is embodied in the UNICEF *Conceptual Framework of Young Child Nutrition* published in 1990.[8] As shown in Figure 1 opposite, the Conceptual Framework brought together in an easily understood manner a practical model that identifies the many key factors causing undernutrition at each level (from the child upwards) across different sectors relevant for nutrition. It also inherently encompasses different viewpoints, including structural and technical dimensions.

Taking the complex problem of undernutrition, the Conceptual Framework clearly communicates how all actors in the nutrition space need to work together to address key causes of undernutrition at each level. The Conceptual Framework's validity today is as great as when it was first published in 1990. It can also be argued that the Conceptual Framework was a quantum leap forward in the way the problem of nutrition has been understood and addressed by the nutrition community. Over time, it has been adapted to include new insights from the growing evidence base of *what we need to do* and *how and when we need to do it*.[9,10]

As shown in Figure1, the *immediate causes* of child undernutrition stem from inadequate dietary intake (e.g. quality and quantity) combined with disease. These are affected in turn by three spheres of *underlying causes*: household food insecurity, inadequate care and feeding practices, and unhealthy environment and inadequate health services, which operate at the family and community level. These three underlying causes are in turn again directly influenced by the basic causes of undernutrition, which include the inadequate financial, human, physical and social capital found in each country. These basic factors are rooted in the overarching sociocultural, economic and political circumstances, and are also often affected by external global factors. Across all dimensions of the Conceptual Framework, it is important to note that the status and access of women to such resources is critical, as women are the nutrition gatekeepers for their children and their families. This is discussed further below.

In summary, undernutrition does not exist in isolation, and it cannot be solved by one sole intervention, as a mix of interventions in different sectors and at different levels is required.

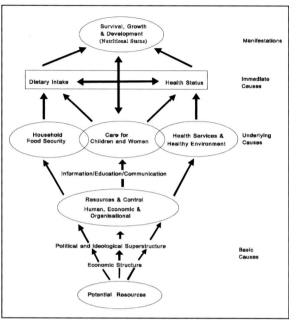

Figure 1: Causes of malnutrition and death.
The original UNICEF Conceptual Framework of Young Child Nutrition
Source: UNICEF Policy Paper (E/ICEF/1990/L.6). Strategy for Improved Nutrition of Children and Women in Developing Countries. ISSN: 1013-3194. Page 22. 9 March 1990.

The need for assessment and analysis before action

Another important consideration is that nutrition problems – and therefore interventions – are highly context-specific. What works in one setting may well not have the desired effects if used without adaptation to a different context. The tendency until the 1990s was to introduce nutrition interventions "lock, stock and barrel," which led to ineffective programs or sometimes to results opposite to those intended.[4] For example, when it was believed that the main cause of malnutrition was protein, some donors spent their resources digging and stocking fish ponds even in areas where fish was in abundant supply. Often no research was carried out to understand the local nutrition circumstances before interventions were designed and rolled out. In fact, it has only been relatively recently that we have had a robust evidence base concerning 'what' nutrition interventions work though we still have much to learn on what can be done to improve nutrition in sectors outside of health. Even in light of these advances, much more attention and investment is still needed to identify cost-effective ways to deliver these proven interventions at scale (e.g. delivery science and the 'how') especially under differing circumstances.

Therefore before any actions are put into place, an *assessment* and *analysis* of the local situation needs to be carried out to inform the design of the actions and ensure their relevance in terms of addressing the actual nutrition problems found in that particular community. This cycle of *Assessment-Analysis-Action*, coined by UNICEF as the Triple A Cycle, is important if we are to understand the immediate factors that affect dietary intake and health status *vis-à-vis* the underlying determinants of household food security, care and feeding practices, and health services including environmental sanitation, as well as higher-level basic factors. While quantitative approaches have their part to play in any process of assessment and analysis, qualitative data are also essential when assessing the nutritional status of a given individual or group, analyzing the findings, and determining the best course of action for improving it. This is in part because many aspects of undernutrition are behavioral, and are better elucidated by means of qualitative rather than quantitative research.

Number of undernourished children today

According to UNICEF (2013), globally more than one quarter (26 percent) of children under 5 years of age were

stunted in 2011. This corresponds to roughly 165 million children worldwide. The burden is not evenly distributed around the world, with sub-Saharan Africa and South Asia being home to three fourths of the world's stunted children. Levels of stunting among children under 5 years of age in sub-Saharan Africa are at 40 percent and in South Asia are at 39 percent. Stunting prevalence is slowly decreasing globally, but in some regions, such as Africa, the absolute number of stunted children is increasing due to high population growth figures. Clearly there is much more work to do.

Latest thinking and the Conceptual Framework

Figure 2 below shows a modified version of the Conceptual Framework which includes the most recent state-of-the-art knowledge from the 2013 Lancet Nutrition Series on what works to improve fetal and child nutrition. Two categories of nutrition actions are shown, nutrition-specific interventions and nutrition-sensitive interventions.[1]

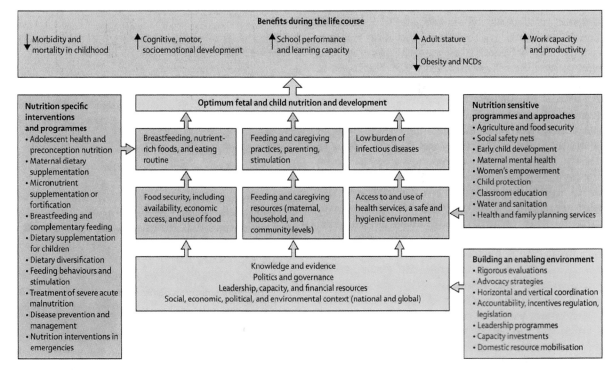

Figure 2: Framework for actions to achieve optimum fetal and child nutrition and development
Source: Black RE, Victora CG, Walker SP, and the Maternal and Child Nutrition Study Group. Maternal and child undernutrition and overweight in low-income and middle-income countries. Figure 1, page 16. The Lancet. 2013.

The definitions of nutrition-specific and nutrition-sensitive are shown in the table, and are discussed further overleaf.

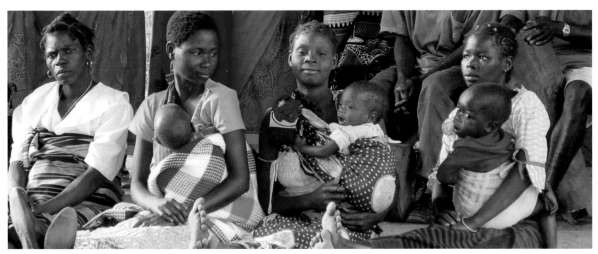

Mozambican mothers and babies
Photo © HKI / Victoria Quinn

Nutrition-specific interventions and programs: Interventions or programs that address the immediate determinants of fetal and child nutrition and development— adequate food and nutrient intake, feeding, caregiving and parenting practices, and low burden of infectious diseases. Examples include:

- adolescent, preconception, and maternal health and nutrition;
- maternal dietary or micronutrient supplementation;
- promotion of optimum breastfeeding;
- promotion of complementary feeding and responsive feeding practices and stimulation;
- dietary supplementation;
- dietary diversification and micronutrient supplementation or fortification for children;
- treatment of severe acute malnutrition;
- disease prevention and management; and
- nutrition in emergencies.

Nutrition-sensitive interventions and programs: Interventions or programs that address the underlying determinants of fetal and child nutrition and development—food security; adequate caregiving resources at the maternal, household and community levels; and access to health services and a safe and hygienic environment—and incorporate specific nutrition goals and actions. Nutrition-sensitive programs can serve as delivery platforms for nutrition-specific interventions, potentially increasing their scale, coverage and effectiveness: Examples include:

- agriculture and food security;
- social safety nets;
- early child development;
- maternal mental health;
- women's empowerment;
- child protection;
- schooling;
- water, sanitation, and hygiene; and
- health and family planning services.

Source: Adapted from Ruel MT, Alderman H, and the Maternal and Child Nutrition Study Group. Nutrition-sensitive interventions and programmes: how can they help to accelerate progress in improving maternal and child nutrition? Page 66. The Lancet. 2013.

Nutrition-specific interventions – proven actions

Nutrition-specific interventions are fairly well-defined due to the solid evidence base that now exists on what actions are proven to make an impact on reducing undernutrition. These nutrition-specific interventions are similar to the set of nutrition actions identified in the original Lancet Maternal and Child Nutrition series published in 2008, and very similar to other approaches including the Essential Nutrition Actions endorsed by other development organizations.[11,12,13]

Apart from needing to know exactly '*what*' to do to improve nutrition at the level of the child or women, it is important to know '*when*' to do it, as the nutrition needs vary throughout their life cycles. Figure 3 below (UNICEF 2013) provides useful programmatic guidance on *what* actions should be promoted *when* during the life cycle of infants, young children and women.

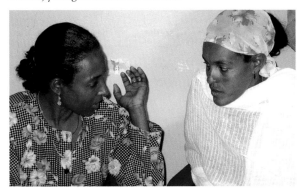

Health worker counseling pregnant woman on early initiation of breastfeeding in Ethiopia
Photo ©: Victoria Quinn

ADOLESCENCE > PREGNANCY	BIRTH	0 – 5 MONTHS	6 – 23 MONTHS
• Improved use of locally available foods	• Early initiation of breastfeeding within one hour of delivery (including colostrum)	• Exclusive breastfeeding	• Timely introduction of adequate, safe and appropriate complementary feeding
• Food fortification, including salt iodization	• Appropriate infant feeding practices for HIV-exposed infants, and antivirals (ARV)	• Appropriate infant feeding practices for HIV-exposed infants, and ARV	• Continued breastfeeding
• Micronutrient supplementation and deworming		• Vitamin A supplementation in first eight weeks after delivery	• Appropriate infant feeding practices for HIV-exposed infants, and ARV
• Fortified food supplements for undernourished mothers		• Multimicronutrient supplementation	• Micronutrient supplementation, including vitamin A, multimicronutrients; zinc treatment for diarrhea; deworming
• Antenatal care, including HIV testing		• Improved use of locally available foods, fortified foods, micronutrient supplementation/home fortification for undernourished women	• Community-based management of severe acute malnutrition; management of moderate acute malnutrition
			• Food fortification, including salt iodization
			• Prevention and treatment of infectious disease; hand washing with soap and improved water and sanitation practices
			• Improved use of locally available foods, fortified foods, micronutrient supplementation/home fortification for undernourished women, hand washing with soap

Figure 3: Key proven practices, services and policy interventions for the prevention and treatment of stunting and other forms of undernutrition throughout the life cycle

Pink refers to interventions for women of reproductive age and mothers. ***Black refers to interventions for young children.***

Source: UNICEF Report "Improving Child Nutrition: The Achievable Imperative for Global Progress. ISBN: 978-92-806-4686-3. Adapted from Figure 2, page 18. 2013. Original sources include: Policy and guideline recommendations based on UNICEF, WHO and other United Nations agencies, Bhutta, Zulfiqar A., et al., 'Maternal and Child Undernutrition 3: What works? Interventions for maternal and child undernutrition and survival', Lancet, vol.371, no.9610, February 2008, pp.417–440.

This nutrition support will sometimes be delivered in the form of counseling (e.g. health worker to mother) to encourage the adoption of optimal nutrition practices (e.g. to give only breast milk during the first six months of her baby's life) or in the form of nutrition supplies (e.g. a health worker providing vitamin A capsules to children starting at six months of age up to 59 months). Behavior change communication, including interpersonal communication, is an important element that needs to be built into the delivery of such nutrition support so that it reaches the right person at the right point in time in the right way. As mentioned earlier, much more attention is needed on 'how' to deliver this nutrition support to vulnerable infants, young children and women at high coverage to have a public health impact.

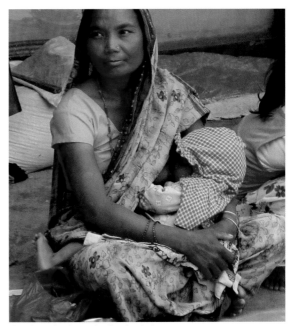

Nepali mother breastfeeding her baby
Photo © HKI / Victoria Quinn

Nutrition-sensitive interventions – still building the evidence base

While undernutrition has a profoundly negative effect on health and well-being, it is not merely a health issue, nor can it be solved only by nutrition-specific interventions confined to the health sector. This is because a range of non-health programs and higher-level policies in other key sectors can also influence nutrition outcomes at broad scale through pathways affecting the underlying and basic causes of undernutrition, especially food, care and health dimensions.

The tendency through the years has been to view undernutrition first and foremost as a health issue, which is likely due to the fact the early work was undertaken by colonial medical doctors as well as nutrition and food scientists studying the effects of deficiencies in protein, vitamins and minerals. However, the fact is that a range of non-health nutrition-sensitive determinants can have a profound effect on nutritional status if they influence the well-being of women, the ability of families to produce or purchase food, maternal and child care and feeding practices or the access of families to adequate health, hygiene and sanitation support. For example, government programs can exert a major impact on nutrition outcomes through such channels as agricultural extension services, consumer and producer food price policies, income and wage policies, and government investments in primary health care and basic education, to name just a few. The status and situation of women throughout is also a critical determinant, especially in terms of how programs may or may not affect their access to essential resources. Even the impact that these programs have on women's use of time can affect nutrition outcomes if they take time away from essential child care, for instance.

Unlike nutrition-specific interventions, nutrition-sensitive development is still being actively debated by global experts, thus a commonly accepted definition has yet to be reached. There is also insufficient evidence on what nutrition-sensitive interventions actually work under what circumstances. Collecting this evidence is a recognized research priority, and would help align our efforts across sectors and at different levels.[14]

More research and documentation regarding what works in terms of agriculture, education, social safety nets, education and programs to reach adolescent girls is needed to build this evidence base.[15] A recent systematic review of agricultural interventions concluded that these did not improve the nutritional status of the children they were targeting. However, the problem is not that agriculture does not have an important effect on nutrition and child growth, but that many of these programs, including the ones studied

in the review above, are poorly designed with weak monitoring and evaluation systems.[15] Better designed programs, including their monitoring and evaluation dimensions, are needed. This will allow us to assess the 'process' aspect of programs, for example, in terms of whether programs are being delivered as originally planned or if other unexpected factors have emerged that have adverse effects on implementation.

Work to this end, especially research, is imperative. As stated in the recent 2013 Lancet series, the *"acceleration of progress in nutrition will require effective, large-scale nutrition-sensitive programmers that address key underlying determinants of nutrition and enhance the coverage and effectiveness of nutrition-specific interventions"*.[15] Lastly, the reach of nutrition-sensitive programs could be immense as they *"…can have a pivotal role in prevention of the excess stunting, wasting, and impaired child development that the scale-up of nutrition-specific interventions cannot resolve on its own"*.[15]

Women are central to the solution

As touched upon above, the role of women in improving child undernutrition and stunting is critical. Not only are mothers key providers for the family, producing much of the food and generating income, but they are also the gatekeepers of their children's nutritional status in their role as caretakers overseeing the feeding, health and hygiene care of their infants and young children. Often the health and nutritional status of women is compromised for a variety of reasons due to past constraints (e.g. long-term results of childhood stunting) and current constraints (e.g. too little food also low in micronutrients, malaria, too many closely spaced pregnancies).

Undernutrition in pregnant women puts newborns at high risk of being born with low birth weight. This in turn leads to an intergenerational cycle where malnourished girls grow to be malnourished women who are at greater risk of giving birth to malnourished babies.[16]

Recent evidence also shows that undernutrition during pregnancy, affecting fetal growth and the first two years of life, is a major determinant not only of stunting, but also of subsequent obesity and non-communicable diseases in adulthood.[1,17,18] Thus undernutrition, overnutrition and non-communicable diseases later in adult life all appear to be interwoven with the sub-optimal development of the fetus in the womb if the pregnant woman herself is suffering from undernutrition.

The long road to food, care and health

In recent years, progress in nutrition has been made on a number of fronts, for example the high coverage of young children with twice yearly supplementation with vitamin A (UNICEF 2013). Unfortunately on many other fronts, including the adoption of optimal breastfeeding and complementary feeding practices, the reduction in acute malnutrition, and the continuing high levels of maternal and child anemia, much more progress is necessary, so there is still much more work to do.

The notion of food, care and health is now widely used today, as is evidenced by global nutrition documents using the Conceptual Framework as the basis on which to develop their nutrition strategies and recommendations.[19] It has also been embraced by the global Scaling Up Nutrition (SUN) Movement, launched in 2010, which comprises many international, regional and national groups committed to taking evidence-based nutrition actions to scale and is discussed extensively elsewhere in this volume. The SUN Movement has made significant progress in recent times, and by mid-2013, the leadership of forty countries from Africa, Asia and Latin America had made commitments to address undernutrition. Half of these countries have also released costed nutrition plans which they intend to roll out to reduce levels of undernutrition. More countries are expected to engage in a similar manner in the coming months. Also, very importantly, in 2012 the World Health Organization (WHO) set global targets to reduce stunting by 40 percent (along with other indicators and targets).[20] With these WHO global targets, our end goal to reduce undernutrition has been clearly spelt out. Achieving this will necessitate continued investment, focus and resolve in the years ahead.

It should be underscored that under the national governments within the SUN Movement are in the driver's seat and are fundamentally responsible for bringing about change via their relevant ministries and departments (the ministries of agriculture, health, and education). Today we know that successfully addressing undernutrition and its various determinants will require strong political will, especially on the part of national governments and leadership. Strong commitment and follow-up by national leaders creates the 'enabling environment' which is necessary for success. Under the SUN Movement this means a 'whole-of-society' approach must be employed to improve nutrition, based on policies which encourage equity, social justice and the empowerment of women.

In addition, close liaison and the sharing of proven best practices between national governments is vital, supported by the agencies of the United Nations. These – UNICEF, WHO, WFP, FAO, IFAD and so on – can play a decisive role in delivering insights, expertise, and tried and tested approaches along with other development partners including civil society, but all must work more closely together, as well as with the national governments they advise. It is to be hoped that the SUN Movement will encourage improved sharing of best practice between governmental and civil society in the service of better nutrition. The private sector and academia – both of which are key players within the SUN Movement – also have an important contribution to make in delivering the nutrition-sensitive actions that will bring about positive change.

None of this, however, is achievable without the necessary human resources and national capacity development in nutrition. In both the health and the relevant non-health sectors, a significant investment must be made in developing a cadre of skilled professionals in key sectors who have improvements in nutrition as explicitly parts of their job descriptions.[21]

Above and beyond this, the world of nutrition has had to respond to a range of developments which lie far beyond its original remit. These include, for instance, the humanitarian crises triggered by natural and man-made disasters (famines, earthquakes, tsunamis, wars), the phenomenon of HIV/AIDS, the spread of non-communicable diseases such as type 2 diabetes and cardiovascular disease, unprecedented population growth, and climate change. Fortunately, the world of nutrition is now united in the first decade of the 21st century through the SUN Movement to promote national action through a global agenda addressing these issues.

The reality, however, is that it will still take time for major inroads to be made to ensure that high enough coverage of vulnerable women and children under two years is achieved with quality nutrition support at critical points in the life cycle so as to make a public health impact. The feeling, and hope, is that we are now on the right path and that the political will needed at all levels but most especially from national leadership and the donor community remains strong and unwavering.

83

Enhanced homestead food production: The view of Helen Keller International (HKI)

The Problem

- Despite significant progress achieved since 1990, according to the Food and Agriculture Organization, today in 2013 one in eight people around the globe still goes hungry every day. The diets of more than one in four are comprised predominantly of staple crops, which, even when they fill the stomach, lack essential vitamins and minerals for health, vitality and survival.

- This global food crisis is worsening the problem of undernutrition across developing regions of the world leading to stunted physical growth and mental development in young children as well as contributing to nearly half of all child deaths worldwide.

- Conditions in various developing nations are particularly severe, and food price volatility is making matters worse for many families, striking rural and urban areas alike.

What HKI Is Doing

- With its partners in government and civil society, since 1988 Helen Keller International (HKI) has been honing a nutrition-sensitive agricultural approach to address these problems. The goal of HKI's Enhanced Homestead Food Production (EHFP) program is to put crops in the ground, nutrients in the diet, and food in the mouths of the most vulnerable family members in communities affected by prolonged undernutrition and food insecurity.

- To date, nearly one million families in Asia (Bangladesh, Cambodia, Indonesia, Nepal and the Philippines) have been reached. The EHFP approach is now being tested and adapted in sub-Saharan Africa in the countries of Burkina Faso, Cote d'Ivoire, Senegal and Tanzania.

- EHFP targets women from poor households with young children as the primary beneficiaries, placing farming inputs, knowledge and skills directly in their hands.

- HKI works in collaboration with local government agriculture and health teams and the staff of non-governmental organizations (NGOs) to develop their capacity to provide long-term support to sustain the activities after three years of external assistance.

- The program helps communities establish technically improved local food production yielding micronutrient-rich fruits and vegetables complemented with poultry and small livestock. This diversified production ensures the year-round availability of vitamins and minerals essential for proper immune system function and full physical, intellectual and cognitive development and which are often lacking in traditional diets.

- EHFP also contains a strong nutrition behavior change component targeting the mothers and other family and community members to ensure not only is more diverse and nutritious food produced but that that food benefits those who need it the most, namely infants and children under two years and pregnant and lacating women. Evidenced-based Essential Nutrition Actions are promoted at each point of the life cycle-from conception to the second year of life-and span the promotion of optimal breastfeeding and complementary feeding, micronutrient consumption, and women's nutrition.

- In Asia where the model was conceived, EHFP has used Village Model Farms (VMF) as a site for community demonstration and training and for the production of inputs to allow households to establish vegetable, pulse and fruit gardens and small animal husbandry (mainly poultry) adjacent to their homesteads. More recently in both Asia and in adaptations for sub-Saharan Africa, HKI has been exploring new approaches to ensure better equity by using a farmer field school model, wherein the demonstration plot is a shared enterprise and female Village Farm Leaders (VFL) are selected for leadership and mentoring skills rather than for having greater resources needed to establish and maintain a private VMF.

- Data collected from EHFP programs across four countries in Asia, where HKI has promoted EHFP the longest, show that households with improved gardens produced on average 45 varieties of vegetables compared to 10 in households with traditional gardens.

- EHFP contributed to significant increases in household income, which was largely invested in improved family well-being, such as education, higher quality foods and productive enterprises. In addition, consumption of dark-green leafy vegetables, orange vegetables and fruits, children's consumption of eggs, and overall household dietary diversity scores increased significantly more in intervention households from baseline to endline compared to controls.

- The prevalence of night blindness (due to vitamin A deficiency) and of anemia has also been shown to be lower in households practicing EHFP.

- In 2009, HKI's Homestead Food Production program in Bangladesh was selected as a case study of a proven nutrition-agriculture model for the International Food Policy Research Institute's "Millions Fed: Proven Successes in Agricultural Development", funded by the Gates Foundation.

Sources: Iannotti, L. et. al. Diversifying into Healthy Diets - Homestead food production in Bangladesh. IFPRI Paper 928. 2009. Campbell, A. et al. Relationship of homestead food production with night blindness among children below 5 years of age in Bangladesh. Public Health Nutr. 2011 Sep;14(9):1627-31. doi: 10.1017/S1368980011000693. Epub May 4 2011. Talukder A, et. al. Homestead food production model contributes to improved household food security and nutrition status of young children and women in poor populations - lessons learned from scaling-up programs in Asia (Bangladesh, Cambodia, Nepal and Philippines). The Journal of Field Actions: Field Actions Science Reports (FACTS Report); Special Issue 2010.

Case study

Scaling up Essential Nutrient Actions in Madagascar

From 1997 to 2006 the Essential Nutrition Actions (ENA) were adapted in Madagascar, through the USAID funded LINKAGES project. ENA provides a framework through which evidenced based nutrition support on infant and young child feeding, micronutrients and women's nutrition can be targeted to children under two years and their mothers at critical life cycle points using existing programs in the health sector.

In 1997 an inter-sectoral nutrition coalition called the *Groupe d'Actions Inter-Sectoriel en Nutrition* was formed with support from USAID, UNICEF and the World Bank. Chaired by the Nutrition Division of the Ministry of Health, the *Groupe d'Actions Inter-Sectoriel en Nutrition* comprised more than 75 representatives from 50 organizations, including government ministries (health, finance, education, agriculture, trade, population) and representatives from the donor community and nongovernmental organizations. Key aspects of this group's work to implement the ENA framework at scale included:

- **Vision:** A shared vision to achieve scale with ENA was established from the very beginning.

- **Wide coverage:** Many partners, especially those with big field programs with wide reach were encouraged to participate, and multiple programs served as opportunities for entry points to implement support for ENA.

- **Specificity:** Initial focus was placed on promoting optimal breastfeeding practices within the overall context of the integrated package of ENAs which also included support to complementary feeding, micronutrients as well as women's nutrition.

- **Harmonization:** Partners reached consensus on ENA messages and field approaches so that everyone was "singing the same nutrition song to the same tune".

- **Support to all levels:** Groups at the national level, regional/district levels, and community level received support.

- **Short-term, skills-based training:** Training modules for health workers and community members included counseling and negotiation skills to encourage mothers and other child caretakers to adopt optimal nutrition behaviors promoted by the ENA framework; these training modules were integrated into existing child survival, reproductive health, and nutrition programs.

- **Behavior change:** A behavior change strategy, based on formative research on local nutrition practices including barriers and obstacles mothers faced, was used to design and promote key ENA messages on small, do-able actions known to make a difference.

- **Community volunteers:** Members of women's groups were trained in ENA promotion and subsequently were able to support health workers stationed at primary facilities in the promotion of optimal nutrition practices.

- **Monitoring and evaluation:** Key ENA indicators and results were collected annually and shared with all partners to celebrate results and encourage success breeding more success.

Through the LINKAGES project, ENA support reached a total of 6.3 million people (out of a total national population of 19 million) in selected program sites. Over a five-year period in these areas, timely initiation of breastfeeding increased from 34 percent to 68 percent, and exclusive breastfeeding increased from 46 percent to 70 percent. The ENA field approach may have spilled over to improve infant and young child feeding practices in non-program sites since at the national level between 1997 and 2003, early initiation of breastfeeding rose from 34 percent to 62 percent, and exclusive breastfeeding increased from 47 percent to 67 percent (2003 Madagascar Demographic Health Survey).

Sources: Quinn VJ, Guyon AB, Schubert JW, Stone-Jimenez MA, Hainsworth M, and Martin L. Improving breastfeeding practices at broad scale at the community level: Success stories from Africa and Latin America. J Hum Lact 21: 345-354. 2005. http://www.linkagesproject.org/ publications/index.php?detail=29 (26 July 2013). Guyon, AB, Quinn, VJ, Hainsworth, M. Ravonimanantsoa, P, Ravelojoana V., Rambeloson, Z, and Martin, L. Implementing an integrated nutrition package at large scale in Madagascar: The Essential Nutrition Actions Framework Food and Nutrition Bulletin, vol. 30, no. 3, The United Nations University. 2009.

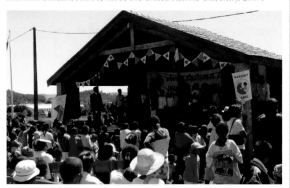

Community mobilization being used in Madagascar to promote optimal breastfeeding practices
Photo © Victoria Quinn

Case study

Why malnutrition persists in many food-secure households

- Mothers have too little time to take care of their young children or themselves during pregnancy.

- Mothers of newborns discard colostrum, the first milk, which strengthens the child's immune system.

- Mothers often feed children under age six months foods other than breast milk even though exclusive breastfeeding is the best source of nutrients and the best protection against many infectious and chronic diseases.

- Caregivers start introducing complementary solid foods too late.

- Caregivers feed children under age two years too little food, or foods that are not energy dense.

- Though food is available, because of inappropriate household food allocation, women and young children's needs are not met and their diets often do not contain enough of the right micronutrients or protein.

- Caregivers do not know how to feed children during and following diarrhea or fever.

- Caregivers' poor hygiene contaminates food with bacteria or parasites.

Source: Directions in Development: Repositioning Nutrition as Central to Development – A Strategy for Large-Scale Action, The International Bank for Reconstruction and Development/The World Bank, 2006.

Three myths about nutrition

Poor nutrition is implicated in more than half of all child deaths worldwide – a proportion unmatched by any infectious disease since the Black Death. It is intimately linked with poor health and environmental factors. But planners, politicians, and economists often fail to recognize these connections.

Serious misapprehensions include the following myths:

Myth 1

Malnutrition is primarily a matter of inadequate food intake. Not so. Food is of course important. But most serious malnutrition is caused by bad sanitation and disease, leading to diarrhea, especially among young children. Women's status and women's education play big parts in improving nutrition. Improving care of young children is vital.

Myth 2

Improved nutrition is a by-product of other measures of poverty reduction and economic advance. It is not possible to jump-start the process. Again, untrue. Improving nutrition requires focused action by parents and communities, backed by local and national action in

health and public services, especially water and sanitation. Thailand has shown that moderate and severe malnutrition can be reduced by 75 percent or more in a decade by such means.

Myth 3

Given scarce resources, broad-based action on nutrition is hardly feasible on a mass scale, especially in poor countries. Wrong again. In spite of severe economic setbacks, many developing countries have made impressive progress. More than two thirds of the people in developing countries now eat iodized salt, combating the iodine deficiency and anemia that affect about 3.5 billion people, especially women and children in some 100 nations. About 450 million children a year now receive vitamin A capsules, tackling the deficiency that causes blindness and increases child mortality. New ways have been found to promote and support breastfeeding, and breastfeeding rates are being maintained in many countries and increased in some. Mass immunization and promotion of oral rehydration to reduce deaths from diarrhea have also done much to improve nutrition.

Source: Directions in Development: Repositioning Nutrition as Central to Development – A Strategy for Large-Scale Action, The International Bank for Reconstruction and Development/The World Bank, 2006 (extracted from Jolly [1996]).

The window of opportunity for addressing undernutrition

The window of opportunity for improving nutrition is small – from before pregnancy through the first two years of life. There is consensus that the damage to physical growth, brain development, and human capital formation that occurs during this one thousand day period is extensive and largely irreversible. Therefore interventions must focus on this window of opportunity. Any investments after this critical period are much less likely to improve nutrition.

The vicious cycle of poverty and malnutrition

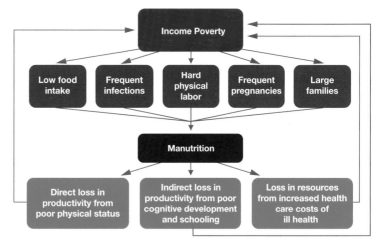

Source: Modified from World Bank (2002a(; Bhagwati and others (2004)

My personal view

Victoria Quinn
Senior Vice President of Programs, Helen Keller International, New York, USA
Adjunct Associate Professor, Friedman School of Nutrition Science and Policy, Boston, USA

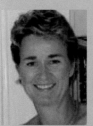

How do we know when we've been successful?

Care must be taken in applying the correct metrics for measuring progress made in reducing undernutrition and hunger. National food balance reports, which have frequently been used in the past to assess these problems, provide a theoretical picture of the food available per capita in a given population and do not necessarily reflect the reality of what goes into people's mouths. The presence of food (especially increasing production levels) is centrally important but does not necessarily ensure the presence of optimal nutrition, as factors such as the quality of food and access of vulnerable groups to purchase or grow it must be considered, along with other factors related to care and health.

Only when children are well nourished and developing in the direction of achieving their full growth potential can we say that our efforts have been successful. Too often, policymakers focus on economic indicators or national agricultural production yields to determine how well a nation is faring. In fact, investments in national and economic development should use the growth of children, particularly stunting, as the best and most accurate yardstick – a human yardstick – to measure success. Indicators of child undernutrition, such as height, reflect much more accurately than gross domestic product whether development and human welfare has truly progressed in a country.

Further reading

UNICEF Policy Paper (E/ICEF/1990/L.6). Strategy for Improved Nutrition of Children and Women in Developing Countries8

World Bank. Repositioning nutrition as central to development: A strategy for large-scale action19

UNICEF. Tracking Progress on Child and Maternal Nutrition: A survival and development priority. New York, NY, USA: UNICEF, 2009

Jonsson, U. Commentary: The Rise and Fall of Paradigms in World Food and Nutrition Policy.3

Horton S, Shekar M, McDonald C et al. Scaling Up Nutrition: What will it Cost? Washington DC, USA: World Bank 2010.

2008 Lancet Series on Maternal and Child Undernutrition

UNICEF Report "Improving Child Nutrition: The Achievable Imperative for Global Progress."9

2013 Lancet Series on Maternal and Child Nutrition

References

1   Black RE, Victora CG, Walker SP, and the Maternal and Child Nutrition Study Group. Maternal and child undernutrition and overweight in low-income and middle-income countries. Lancet 2013;382:427–451.

2. Prado E, Dewey K. Nutrition and brain development in early life. Alive and Thrive Technical Brief 2012; Issue 4.

3. Jonsson U. The rise and fall of paradigms in world food and nutrition policy. (Commentary). World Nutrition 2010;1(3):128–158.

4. Quinn V. Nutrition and National Development: An evaluation of nutrition planning in Malawi from 1936 to 1990. The Hague, The Netherlands: Wageningen Agricultural University Press 1994.

5. McLaren D. The Great Protein Fiasco. Lancet 1974;7872:93–96.

6. Berg A. (1987). Nutrition Planning is Alive and Well, Thank You. Food Policy 1987; 12(4):365–375. Rejoinder to: Field JO. (1987). Multisectoral Nutrition Planning: A Post-Mortem. Food Policy 1987;12(1):15–28.

7. UNICEF 1993, "We Shall Never Go Back"

8. UNICEF Policy Paper (E/ICEF/1990/L.6). Strategy for Improved Nutrition of Children and Women in Developing Countries. New York, NY, USA: UNICEF, 1990 p.22.

9. UNICEF. Improving Child Nutrition: The Achievable Imperative for Global Progress. New York, NY, USA: UNICEF, 2013, p.18.

10. Bhutta, ZA, Ahmed T, Black RE et al. What works? Interventions for maternal and child undernutrition and survival. Lancet 2008;371(9610):417–440.

11. USAID. Child Survival Programs – Technical Reference Materials: Nutrition 2006

12. WHO. Essential nutrition actions: improving maternal, newborn, infant and young child health and nutrition. Geneva, Switzerland: World Health Organization, 2013.

13. Core Group. Essential Nutrition Actions Training Materials. 2011 http://www.coregroup.org

14. Mucha N. Implementing Nutrition-Sensitive Development: Reaching Consensus. Briefing Paper. Washington DC, USA: Bread for the World, 2012

15. Ruel MT, Alderman H, and the Maternal and Child Nutrition Study Group. Nutrition-sensitive interventions and programmes: how can they help to accelerate progress in improving maternal and child nutrition? Lancet 2013;382(9891):536–551

16. Özaltin E, Hill K, Subramanian SV. Association of maternal stature with offspring mortality, underweight, and stunting in low- to middle-income countries. JAMA 2010;303(15):1507–1516;

17. Barker DJP. Maternal Nutrition, Fetal Nutrition, and Disease in Later Life. Nutrition 1997;13(9):807–813

18. Uauy R, Kain J, Corvalan C. How Can the Developmental Origin of Health and Disease [DOHaD] Hypothesis Contribute to Improving Health in Developing Countries? Am J Clin Nutr 2011;94(6):1759S.

19. World Bank. Repositioning Nutrition as Central to Development: A Strategy for Large-Scale Action. Washington, DC, USA: World Bank, 2006.

20. WHO Comprehensive Implementation Plan on Maternal, Infant and Young Child Nutrition, endorsed by the 65th World Health Assembly, May 2012

21. Mucha N, Tharaney M. Strengthening Human Capacity to Scale Up Nutrition. Report by Bread for the World and Helen Keller International, June 2013

Chapter Seven

How to Improve Nutrition via Effective Programming

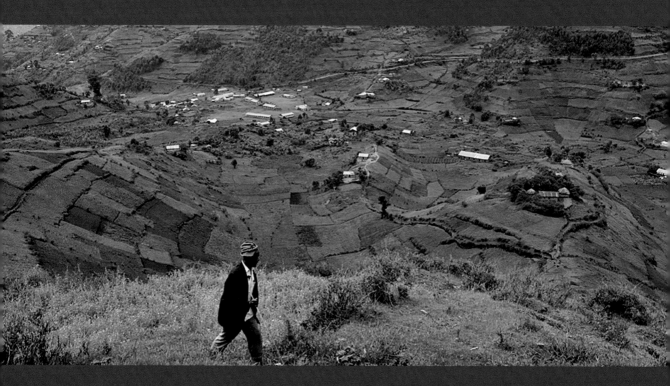

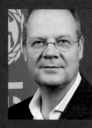

Werner Schultink

Associate Director,
UNICEF

Key messages

- Reductions in stunting and other forms of undernutrition can be achieved through proven interventions. These include improving women's nutrition, especially before, during and after pregnancy; early and exclusive breastfeeding; timely, safe, appropriate and high-quality complementary food; and appropriate micronutrient interventions.

- Timing is important – interventions should focus on the critical 1,000-day window including pregnancy and before a child turns two. After that window closes, disproportionate weight gain may increase the child's risk of becoming overweight and developing health problems such as non-communicable diseases in adult life.

- Efforts to scale up nutrition programs are working, benefiting women and children and their communities in many countries. Such programs all have common elements: political commitment, national policies and programs based on sound evidence and analysis, the presence of trained and skilled community workers collaborating with communities, effective communication and advocacy, and multi-sectoral, integrated service delivery.

UNICEF's 2009 report Tracking Progress on Child and Maternal Nutrition drew attention to the impact of high levels of undernutrition on child survival, growth and development and their social and economic toll on nations. It described the state of nutrition programs worldwide and argued for improving and expanding delivery of key nutrition interventions during the critical 1,000-day window covering a woman's pregnancy and the first two years of her child's life, when rapid physical and mental development occurs. This chapter builds on those earlier findings by highlighting new developments and demonstrating that efforts to scale up nutrition programs are working, benefiting children in many countries. It is based on the 2013 UNICEF publication Improving Child Nutrition: The achievable imperative for global progress.

Nutrition-specific interventions

Nutrition-specific interventions are actions that have a direct impact on the prevention and treatment of undernutrition, in particular during the 1,000 days covering pregnancy and the child's first two years. These interventions should be complemented by broader, nutrition-sensitive approaches that have an indirect impact on nutrition status. Equity considerations in nutrition programming are particularly important, as stunting and other forms of undernutrition usually afflict the most vulnerable populations.

Promoting optimal nutrition practices, meeting micronutrient requirements and preventing and treating severe acute malnutrition are key goals for nutrition programming. The 2009 Tracking Progress on Child and Maternal Nutrition report summarized the evidence base for nutrition-specific interventions.

Key proven practices, services and policy interventions for the prevention and treatment of stunting and other forms of undernutrition throughout the life cycle

Adolescence to Pregnancy	Birth	0 to 5 Months	6 to 23 Months
⊕ Improved use of locally available foods	+ Early initiation of breastfeeding within one hour of delivery (including colostrum)	+ Exclusive breastfeeding	+ Timely introduction of adequate, safe and appropriate complementary feeding
⊕ Food fortification, including salt iodization	+ Appropriate infant feeding practices for HIV-exposed infants, and antivirals (ARV)	+ Appropriate infant feeding practices for HIV-exposed infants, and ARV	+ Continued breastfeeding
⊕ Micronutrient supplementation and deworming		⊕ Vitamin A supplementation in first eight weeks after delivery	+ Appropriate infant feeding practices for HIV-exposed infants, and ARV
⊕ Fortified food supplements for undernourished mothers		⊕ Multi-micronutrient supplementation	+ Micronutrient supplementation, including vitamin A, multi-micronutrients; zinc treatment for diarrhoea; deworming
⊕ Antenatal care, including HIV testing		⊕ Improved use of locally available foods, fortified foods, micronutrient supplementation/home fortification for undernourished women	+ Community-based management of severe acute malnutrition; management of moderate acute malnutrition
			+ Food fortification, including salt iodization
			+ Prevention and treatment of infectious disease; hand washing with soap and improved water and sanitation practices
			⊕ Improved use of locally available foods, fortified foods, micronutrient supplementation/home fortification for undernourished women, hand washing with soap

Key:
⊕ **interventions for women of reproductive age and mothers.**
+ **interventions for young children.**

Source: Policy and guideline recommendations based on UNICEF, WHO and other United Nations agencies, Bhutta ZA, Ahmed T, Black RE et al. 'Maternal and Child Undernutrition 3: What works? Interventions for maternal and child undernutrition and survival', Lancet, vol. 371, no. 9610, February 2008, pp. 417–440, derived from 2013 UNICEF publication Improving Child Nutrition: The achievable imperative for global progress

Taking a life-cycle approach, the activities fall broadly into the following categories:

• Maternal nutrition and prevention of low birth weight

• Infant and young child nutrition (IYCN)

   – Breastfeeding, with early initiation (within one hour of birth) and continued exclusive breastfeeding for the first six months followed by continued breastfeeding up to 2 years

   – Safe, timely, adequate and appropriate complementary feeding from 6 months onwards

• Prevention and treatment of micronutrient deficiencies

• Prevention and treatment of severe acute malnutrition

• Promotion of good sanitation practices and access to clean drinking water

• Promotion of healthy practices and appropriate use of health services

Maternal nutrition

Nutritional status before and during pregnancy influences maternal and child health. Optimal child development requires adequate nutrient intake, provision of supplements as needed, and prevention of disease. It also requires protection from stress factors such as cigarette smoke, narcotic substances, environmental pollutants and psychological stress. Maternal malnutrition leads to poor fetal growth and low birth weight.

Interventions to improve maternal nutrient intake include supplementation with iron, folic acid, iodine, or multiple micronutrients and provision of food and other supplements where necessary. Compared to iron-folic acid supplementation alone, supplementation with multiple micronutrients during pregnancy has been found to reduce low birth weight by about 10 percent in low-income countries. Adequate intake of folic acid and iodine around conception and of iron and iodine during pregnancy are important, especially for development of the infant's brain.

Among undernourished women, balanced protein-energy supplementation has been found effective in reducing the prevalence of low birth weight. The use of lipid-based supplements for pregnant women in emergency settings is being studied as a way to improve child growth and development.

Many interventions to promote maternal health and fetal growth are delivered by the health system and through community-based programs. Antenatal care visits should be used to promote optimal nutrition and deliver specific interventions, such as malaria prophylaxis and treatment and deworming. Community-based education and communication programs can encourage appropriate behaviors to improve nutrition.

Beyond such specific interventions, other relevant interventions include preventing pregnancy during adolescence, delaying age of marriage, preventing unwanted or unplanned pregnancy, increased birth spacing and overcoming sociocultural barriers to healthy practices and healthcare-seeking.

Early initiation of breastfeeding

Several studies have demonstrated that early initiation of breastfeeding reduces the risk of neonatal mortality. Colostrum, the rich milk produced by the mother during the first few days after delivery, provides essential nutrients as well as antibodies to boost the baby's immune system, thus reducing the likelihood of death in the neonatal period. Beyond saving lives, early initiation of breastfeeding promotes stronger uterine contractions, reducing the likelihood of uterine bleeding. It also reduces the risk of hypothermia, improves bonding between mother and child and promotes early milk production.

Fewer than half of newborns globally are put to the breast within the first hour of birth, though early initiation of breastfeeding is higher in least-developed countries (52 percent in 2011).

Exclusive breastfeeding

Exclusive breastfeeding in the first six months of life saves lives. During this period, an infant who is not breastfed is more than 14 times more likely to die from all causes than an exclusively breastfed infant. Infants who are exclusively breastfed are less likely to die from diarrhea and pneumonia, the two leading killers of children under 5. Moreover, many other benefits are associated with exclusive breastfeeding for both mother and infant, including prevention of growth faltering.

Globally 39 percent of infants less than 6 months of age were exclusively breastfed in 2011 (Figure 20 ##in original – please renumber for this publication##). Some 76 percent of infants continued to be breastfed at 1 year of age, while only 58 percent continued through the recommended

Globally, less than 40 per cent of infants are exclusively breastfed

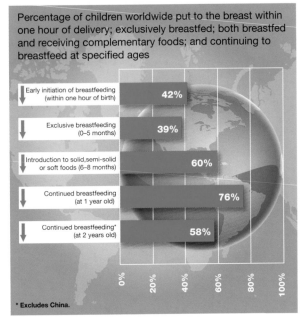

Percentage of children worldwide put to the breast within one hour of delivery; exclusively breastfed; both breastfed and receiving complementary foods; and continuing to breastfeed at specified ages

* Excludes China.

UNICEF Global Nutrition Database, 2012, based on MICS, DHS and other national surveys, 2007–2011.

Most regions have increased rates of exclusive breastfeeding

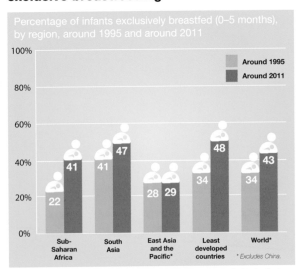

Percentage of infants exclusively breastfed (0–5 months), by region, around 1995 and around 2011

Note: Estimates based on a subset of 50 countries with available trend data. Regional estimates are presented only where adequate population coverage is met. Rates around 2011 may differ from current rates, as trend analysis is based on a subset of countries.

UNICEF Global Nutrition Database, 2012, based on MICS, DHS and other national surveys.

duration of up to two years. The regions with the highest exclusive breastfeeding rates of infants under 6 months old were Eastern and Southern Africa (52 percent) and South Asia (47 percent), with similar rates in least-developed countries as a whole. However, coverage is lowest in sub-Saharan Africa, with 37 percent of infants less than 6 months of age exclusively breastfed in 2011. This is due largely to the low rate in West and Central Africa (25 percent) compared to Eastern and Southern Africa (52 percent).

Rates of exclusive breastfeeding have increased by more than 20 percent, from 34 percent around 1995 to 43 percent around 2011. It is particularly encouraging to note the nearly 50 percent increase in exclusive breastfeeding rates in sub-Saharan Africa, from 22 percent to 41 percent during this period. Progress has also been made in least developed countries, where exclusive breastfeeding rates increased by nearly one third, from 34 percent to 48 percent.

Complementary feeding

Studies have shown that feeding with appropriate, adequate and safe complementary foods from the age of 6 months onwards leads to better health and growth of children. Breast milk remains an important source of nutrients, and it is recommended that breastfeeding continue until children reach 2 years of age. In vulnerable populations especially, good complementary feeding practices have been shown to reduce stunting markedly and rapidly.

Key principles guide programming for complementary feeding. They include education to improve caregiver practices; increasing energy density and/ or nutrient bioavailability of

complementary foods; providing complementary foods, with or without added micronutrients; and fortifying complementary foods, either centrally or through home fortification including use of multiple micronutrient powder (MNP), in each case paying greater attention to food-insecure populations.

Globally, only 60 percent of children aged 6 to 8 months receive solid, semi-solid or soft foods, highlighting deficiencies in the timely introduction of complementary foods. Of the 24 countries profiled in this report, only 8 had recent data reflecting both the frequency and quality of complementary feeding for children aged 6 to 23 months.

Complementary feeding in eight countries

Percentage of breastfed and non-breastfed children aged 6–23 months receiving minimum acceptable diet, minimum dietary diversity, and minimum meal frequency

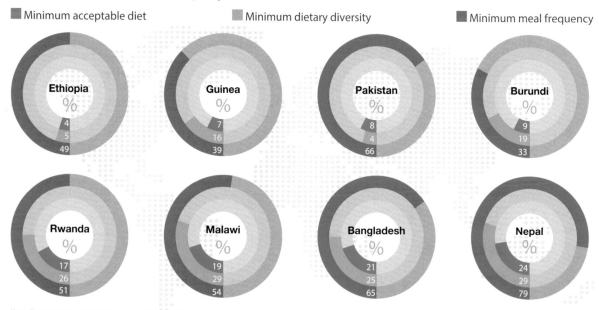

Note: The eight countries selected were those profiled in this report with available data on complementary feeding indicators. Minimum meal frequency refers to the percentage of children aged 6–23 months who received solid, semi-solid or soft foods the minimum number of times or more (for breastfed children, minimum is defined as two times for infants 6–8 months and three times for children 9–23 months; for non-breastfed children, minimum is defined as four times for children 6–23 months); minimum dietary diversity refers to the percentage of children aged 6–23 months who received foods from four or more food groups; and minimum acceptable diet refers to the percentage of children aged 6–23 months who received a minimum acceptable diet both in terms of frequency and quality, apart from breastmilk.

UNICEF Global Nutrition Database, 2012, based on MICS, DHS and other national surveys, 2010–2012.

93

Many countries have increased rates of exclusive breastfeeding

Percentage of infants exclusively breastfed (0–5 months), by country, around 1995 and around 2011

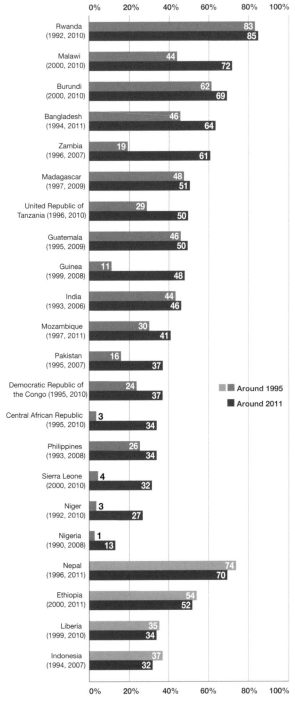

Infant and Young Child Nutrition (IYCN)

Optimal IYCN practices include initiating breastfeeding within one hour of birth, exclusive breastfeeding for the first six months of life and continued breastfeeding up to the age of 2 and beyond, together with safe, age-appropriate feeding of solid, semi-solid and soft food starting at 6 months of age.

Two practices together – ensuring optimal breastfeeding in the first year and complementary feeding practices – could prevent almost one fifth of deaths of children under 5 years of age. Studies suggest that optimal breastfeeding improves brain development. Breastfeeding may also protect against cardiovascular risk factors, although it is not yet clear whether this is the case in low- and middle-income settings.

Nutrition programming in this area continues to receive insufficient attention, despite the well-established benefits of age-appropriate IYCN practices. Valuable lessons from programming experiences have led to changes to IYCN strategies. A comprehensive, multi-pronged approach is needed, with both cross-cutting and targeted strategies at community, health system and national levels.

Key components and interventions of an infant and young child feeding strategy

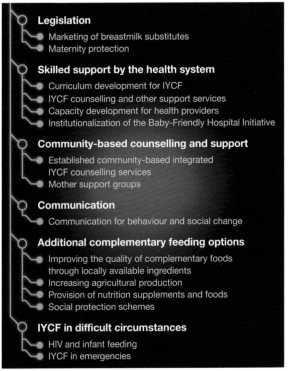

Legislation
- Marketing of breastmilk substitutes
- Maternity protection

Skilled support by the health system
- Curriculum development for IYCF
- IYCF counselling and other support services
- Capacity development for health providers
- Institutionalization of the Baby-Friendly Hospital Initiative

Community-based counselling and support
- Established community-based integrated IYCF counselling services
- Mother support groups

Communication
- Communication for behaviour and social change

Additional complementary feeding options
- Improving the quality of complementary foods through locally available ingredients
- Increasing agricultural production
- Provision of nutrition supplements and foods
- Social protection schemes

IYCF in difficult circumstances
- HIV and infant feeding
- IYCF in emergencies

Adapted from Programming Guide: Infant and young child feeding, UNICEF, 2011.

Continuing the Discussion on Adequate Nutrient Intakes for Infancy

The following letter by Zulfiqar Ahmed Bhutta, which appeared in Sight and Life *magazine, Vol. 27 (1) 2013, is a response to David Thurnham's article on "Adequate Nutrient Intakes for Infancy, Part 1: From 0 to 6 Months," published in* Sight and Life *magazine, Vol. 26 (3) 2012 [Ed.]*

The article by Thurnham[1] in *Sight and Life* 3/2012 reviews the evidence around breast milk volumes, nutrient composition and recommendations for infants under six months of age. The review covers a vast landscape and summarizes pertinent information as to volume, energy and micronutrient needs, and adequacy of intake through breastfeeding and breast milk. In addition to useful information on milk volumes and energy, an important conclusion made by the authors is the identification of Group 2 nutrients whose concentrations are unaffected by maternal intake, and can lead to maternal depletion. This is a key step in addressing the adequacy of intake in the first six months of life.

The review highlights two areas that merit further work. Firstly, there exists a real need to develop sensitive and reliable methods for estimating breast milk intake in a range of settings. The continued reliance on test-weighing and the variability in measurements in ambulatory settings makes this a less-than-optimal method for assessing breast milk volume. Although there are established stable isotope techniques for measuring breast milk intake[2,3] these are onerous and not widely available. Secondly, information on breast milk intake and quality in malnourished populations is also outdated, and few studies have been conducted in populations with high rates of HIV infection or among wasted women with a body mass index <18.5. While studies do suggest that the volume of breast milk produced may not be affected during acute infection, milk composition is known to change during this state.[4] Although the effects of marginal maternal malnutrition on breast milk composition and quality are well-recognized,[5] these effects may be exaggerated among populations with more severe forms of maternal wasting and concomitant infections such as HIV.

Investments must be made in optimizing the health and nutrition of mothers

As underscored by Thurnham et al,[1] the onset of linear growth failure among young infants varies in different populations. While the onset of stunting may accompany the introduction of complementary foods after 4–6 months, and coincidental infections,[6] in many regions the onset of linear growth retardation may occur earlier[7] and reflect the impact of maternal health factors and micronutrient deficiencies. The implications of these findings and the limitations of addressing key micronutrient deficiencies sufficiently through maternal supplementation during lactation suggest the need for intervening early during pregnancy or the pre-pregnancy period. In many populations with high rates of maternal micronutrient deficiencies and malnutrition, most women present for antenatal care well into the second trimester, and replenishing deficits in this limited time window of pregnancy may not be possible.[8] In such circumstances, reaching adolescent girls and women in the pre-pregnancy period, along with adequate birth-preparedness and nutrition support, is critical in addressing key micronutrient deficits during pregnancy and early infancy. With the increased emphasis on lactation support and counseling for breastfeeding, comparable investments must be made in optimizing the health and nutrition of mothers prior to, and during, pregnancy.

Zulfiqar Ahmed Bhutta

The Noodin Noormahomed Sheriff Endowed Professor and Founding Chair, Division of Women and Child Health, Aga Khan University, Karachi, Pakistan

References

1. Thurnham D. Adquate Micronutrient Intakes for Infancy. Sight and Life Magazine 2012;3:28–39.

2. Wells JC, Jonsdottir OH, Hibberd PL et al. Randomized controlled trial of 4 compared with 6 months of exclusive breastfeeding in Iceland: differences in breast milk intake by stable-isotope probe. Am J Clin Nutr 2012;96:73–9.

3. da Costa TH, Haisma H, Wells JC et al. How much human milk do infants consume? Data from 12 countries using a standardized stable isotope methodology. J Nutr 2010;140:2227–32.

4. Zavaleta N, Lanata C, Butron B et al. Effect of acute maternal infection on quantity and composition of breast milk. Am J Clin Nutr 1995;62:559–63.

5. Brown KH, Akhtar NA, Robertson AD, Ahmed MG. Lactational capacity of marginally nourished mothers: relationships between maternal nutritional status and quantity and proximate composition of milk. Pediatrics 1986;78:909–19.

6. Dewey KG, Peerson JM, Heinig MJ et al. Growth patterns of breast-fed infants in affluent (United States) and poor (Peru) communities: implications for timing of complementary feeding. Am J Clin Nutr 1992;56:1012–8.

7. Victora CG, de Onis M, Hallal PC et al. Worldwide timing of growth faltering: revisiting implications for interventions. Pediatrics. 2010;125:e473–80.

8. Bhutta ZA. Summary on Micronutrient Requirements and Deficiencies in Maternal and Child Nutrition. In Bhutta ZA, Hurrell RF, Rosenberg IH (eds): Meeting Micronutrient Requirements for Health and Development. Nestlé Nutr Inst Workshop Ser Nestec Ltd, Vevey / Basel, Switzerland: S Karger AG 2012;70:74–77.

Prevention and treatment of micronutrient deficiencies

Micronutrient deficiencies, including deficiencies of vitamin A, iron, iodine, zinc and folic acid, are common among women and children in low- and middle-income countries. Ensuring adequate micronutrient status in women of reproductive age, pregnant women and children improves the health of expectant mothers, the growth and development of unborn children, and the survival and physical and mental development of children up to 5 years old.

Programs to address micronutrient deficiencies include delivery of supplements to specific vulnerable groups, home fortification of complementary food for children aged 6 to 23 months and fortification of staple foods and condiments.

Vitamin A supplementation

Globally, one in three preschool-aged children and one in six pregnant women are deficient in vitamin A due to inadequate dietary intake (1995–2005, WHO: http://whqlibdoc.who.int/publications/2009/9789241598019_eng.pdf). The highest prevalence remains in Africa and South-East Asia. Vitamin A is necessary to support immune system response, and children who are deficient face a higher risk of dying from infectious diseases such as measles and diarrhea. Vitamin A supplementation delivered periodically to children aged 6 to 59 months has been shown to be highly effective in reducing mortality (on average -24 percent) from all causes in countries where vitamin A deficiency is a public health problem.

Vitamin A supplementation reaches more than 80 per cent of young children in least developed countries

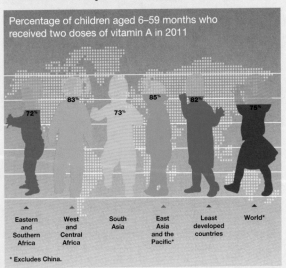

Percentage of children aged 6–59 months who received two doses of vitamin A in 2011

72%	Eastern and Southern Africa
83%	West and Central Africa
73%	South Asia
85%	East Asia and the Pacific*
82%	Least developed countries
75%	World*

* Excludes China.

Source: UNICEF Global Nutrition Databases, 2012. Regional estimates are presented only where adequate population coverage is met.

Globally, three in four children (75 percent) aged 6 to 59 months received two doses of vitamin A in 2011, sufficient to reduce under-five child mortality. Coverage of vitamin A supplementation was highest in East Asia and the Pacific (85 percent; excluding China for lack of data) and West and Central Africa (83 percent). Nearly half of countries reporting these data in 2011 did not reach the 80 percent coverage target.

Iron supplementation

Iron deficiency predominantly affects children, adolescent girls and menstruating and pregnant women. Globally, the most significant contributor to the onset of anemia is iron deficiency. Consequences of iron deficiency include reduced school performance in children and decreased work productivity in adults. Anemia is most prevalent in Africa and Asia, especially among poor populations. Global estimates from the WHO database suggest that about 42 percent of pregnant women and 47 percent of preschool-aged children suffer from anemia.

Universal salt iodization

Iodine deficiency is the most common cause of preventable mental impairment. Fortification of salt is widely used to avert consequences associated with this deficiency. Significant progress has been made in reducing the number of countries whose populations suffer mild to severe iodine deficiency, from 54 countries in 2003 to 32 in 2011. During this period the number of countries reaching adequate iodine intake increased by more than one third, from 43 to 69.

Globally, 75 percent of households have adequately iodized salt (15 parts per million or more), but coverage varies considerably by region. East Asia and the Pacific had the highest coverage, 87 percent in 2011, and as a region had nearly reached the universal salt iodization target of 90 percent. Coverage was lowest in sub-Saharan Africa, where less than half of households have adequately iodized salt. Coverage is generally higher among richer households than poorer households.

One fifth of countries reporting in 2011 had reached the 90 percent target of universal salt iodization. Most had reached only 50 to 70 percent coverage. Support of national salt iodization programs is needed, along with advocacy to increase awareness among country policy-makers about the need to eliminate iodine deficiency, private-public partnerships to assist salt producers with sustained iodization, and education of civil society to build demand for iodized salt.

Iodized salt consumption is more likely among the richest households than the poorest households

Consumption of adequately iodized salt among the richest households compared to the poorest, in countries with available data

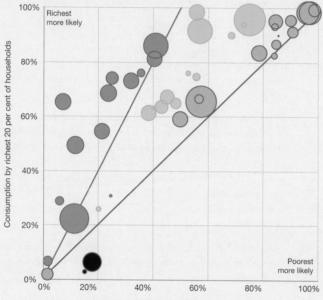

- ● Richest 20% more than twice as likely as poorest 20% (12 countries)
- ○ Richest 20% more likely than poorest 20% (13 countries)
- ● Richest 20% equally as likely as poorest 20% (16 countries)
- ● Richest 20% less likely than poorest 20% (2 countries)

How to read this graph:

Each circle represents data from one country. The size of a circle is proportional to the size of the country's population. The horizontal axis represents the percentage of the poorest 20 per cent of households consuming adequately iodized salt, while the vertical axis represents the percentage of the richest 20 per cent of households. Circles along the green line represent countries in which the likelihood of consuming adequately iodized salt is similar among the richest and the poorest households. Circles above or below the green line suggest disparity. The closeness of circles to the upper-left corner indicates greater advantage for the richest households in that country (greater disadvantage for the poorest households).

Note: Based on 43 countries with available disparity data.

Source: UNICEF Global Nutrition Database, 2012, MICS, DHS and other national surveys, with additional analysis by UNICEF, 2006–2011, derived from 2013 UNICEF publication Improving Child Nutrition: The achievable imperative for global progress.

(chart axis labels: Richest more likely; Poorest more likely; y-axis "Consumption by richest 20 per cent of households" 0%–100%; x-axis "Consumption by poorest 20 per cent of households" 0%–100%)

Fortification of complementary foods, staple foods and condiments

Home fortification

Multiple micronutrient powders (MNPs) offer a low-cost, highly acceptable way to improve the quality of complementary foods. MNPs have been found highly effective in preventing iron deficiency and iron-deficiency anemia. Combined with additional supplementary energy, protein and fats, MNPs have also been shown to improve child growth and development.

Based on a global assessment carried out in 2011, some 22 countries, mostly in Asia and Latin America and the Caribbean, were implementing MNP interventions to improve the quality of complementary food. They reached over 12 million children in 2010, mainly by distributing MNPs through the public health system. Four countries are implementing national-scale programs and 17 countries are working to scale up to a national level. Further expansion is taking place, mainly in Africa and South-East Asia.

Large-scale fortification

Adding micronutrients to staple foods such as wheat and maize flour, cooking oil, sugar, salt, complementary foods and condiments in factories and other production sites is a cost-effective way to improve the micronutrient status of populations. For example, flour is commonly fortified with iron, zinc, folic acid and other B vitamins such as thiamin, riboflavin, niacin, vitamin B12 and vitamin A in some countries. As of December 2012, wheat flour fortification is mandated by law in 75 countries compared with only 33 countries in 2004. The amount of flour currently fortified represents about 30 percent of the global production of wheat flour from industrial mills.

Scaling up nutrition

Kenya continues to shine in addressing malnutrition, a public health problem that also hinders economic development in many developing countries. This week [in November 2012], leaders, professionals, private sector representatives and other partners gathered in Nairobi for a high-level symposium on Scaling Up Nutrition (SUN).

Kenya is one of 31 countries to join the Movement to date. The SUN event comes on the heels of the launch of an exciting public-private partnership, expected to reach 27 million Kenyans with a range of foods fortified with essential vitamins and minerals (micronutrients).

Children who are well-nourished – especially in the 1,000 days between pregnancy and the second birthday – grow up to learn more, earn more and stay healthy. But those who are malnourished suffer irreversible and lifelong damage, including stunted growth and impaired cognitive development.

Based on this evidence, SUN partners focus on implementing solutions that improve nutrition, including support for breastfeeding and ensuring access to essential vitamins and minerals through supplementation, micronutrient powders and food fortification. Countries working to scale up nutrition have established targets tailored to address their own specific challenges and capitalize on their greatest opportunities for lasting impact.

In Kenya, 35 percent of children under five are stunted and over 10 million people suffer from poor nutrition and chronic food insecurity.

Lost productivity

Micronutrient deficiencies are widespread, leading to health problems including blindness, lost productivity, pregnancy complications and increased risk of death from diseases like measles and diarrhea. The Government of Kenya has developed a comprehensive National Food Security and Nutrition Policy and Strategy that recognizes the need for multi-public and private-sector involvement in addressing malnutrition.

They also have a long history of supporting food fortification. The fortification of common foods is a proven, cost-effective way to improve the health and productivity of whole populations. The fortification of commercially produced staple foods continuously delivers nutrients to large segments of the population, without requiring that they change their eating habits.

The impact is huge. Take the case of fortified flour, now required by 57 countries. Fortifying flour with folic acid has reduced cases of brain and spine birth defects (also known as neural tube defects) by up to 70 percent.

The return on investment from micronutrient provision, including food fortification, is astounding. According to the 2012 Copenhagen Consensus panel of experts, every $1 spent providing essential micronutrients to preschoolers generates $30 in benefits. Just last month, the Kenya National Food Fortification Alliance launched the national fortification logo *kuboresha afya* (improving health), marking for Kenyan consumers the range of foods now fortified with vital micronutrients.

If we are going to improve global health and development, we need to scale up nutrition. Proven, high-impact, low-cost interventions like food fortification exist. We need more public-private partnerships to implement these interventions. We need more countries like Kenya to join the SUN, to both share what they have learnt and to learn from other Movement members. Because we can do far more by working together than any one of us could do alone.

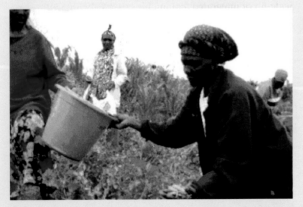

Klaus Kraemer and Gladys Mugambi, www.africareview.com, 9 November 2012 (abridged)
Source: Dr Klaus Kraemer is the Director of Sight and Life, a non-profit humanitarian nutrition think tank of DSM, which cares about the world's most vulnerable populations and exists to help improve their nutritional status.
Gladys Mugambi is Kenya's deputy head of the Division of Nutrition, Food Fortification Project Manager for the Ministry of Public Health and Sanitation, and Secretary of the Kenya National Food Fortification Alliance.

Community-based interventions

Children with severe acute malnutrition (SAM) are nine times more likely to die than children who are well-nourished. Children who are wasted, have highly variable weight-for-height or experience negative changes in weight-for-height, are at a higher risk for linear growth retardation and stunting.

While prevention is the first step towards management of SAM, once it occurs, urgent action is needed to minimize complications and avoid the risk of death. It is increasingly recognized that SAM is a problem not only in emergency contexts but also in non-emergency settings.

Community-based management of acute malnutrition (CMAM) has proven to be successful in treating acute malnutrition and was officially endorsed by the United Nations in 2007. It decentralizes the management of SAM, making it easier to reach and treat children in their communities. It involves early detection of children with SAM with treatment in the community, timely referral to inpatient care for those who need it and subsequent follow-up in the community. Multiple partners have supported this approach in both emergency and non-emergency settings by guiding policy change, providing technical support and making commitments to provide therapeutic supplies. Using this approach, more than 75 percent of treated children are expected to recover. In addition, more children have access to treatment because hospitalization is not required for the majority of cases.

Five countries account for more than half of admissions for treatment of severe acute malnutrition

Number of reported cases admitted for treatment of SAM in 2011

Ethiopia	302,000
Niger	299,000
Somalia	167,000
Pakistan	157,000
Democratic Republic of the Congo	157,000
Total	1,082,000

Note: Figures are presented to the nearest 1,000. There is no standardized system of national reporting, therefore the mode of each country's data collection differs (whether based on health facilities with functional services for SAM or numbers of implementing partners submitting reports). Also note that while Niger, Somalia and Pakistan received 100 per cent of expected reports for 2011, Ethiopia and the Democratic Republic of the Congo indicated receiving 80 per cent of expected reports.

Source: UNICEF Global Nutrition Database, based on Global SAM Update, 2012.

Globally in 2011, an estimated 2 million children under 5 were admitted for treatment of SAM – compared with just over 1 million reported during 2009. This increase in reported admissions is not only indicative of improved access to SAM management, but also reflects improved national reporting.

Key strategies to expand access to quality treatment of SAM include creating national policies to help governments accelerate and sustain scale-up, building national capacities and strengthening systems to support CMAM scale-up, and integrating CMAM into other health and nutrition activities.

Water, sanitation and hygiene and access to health services

Repeated episodes of diarrhea, intestinal infestation with nematode worms and possibly tropical or environmental enteropathy (in which fecal contamination causes changes to the intestines affecting permeability and absorption) can impede nutrient absorption and diminish appetite, resulting in stunting and other forms of undernutrition.

Improving water, sanitation and hygiene as well as housing and access to and use of health services can promote healthy environments and reduce the prevalence of infectious diseases, and key interventions implemented at scale can reduce undernutrition. These include immunization, improving sanitation by creating environments free of open defecation, hand washing with soap, access to clean drinking water, use of oral rehydration salts and therapeutic zinc to treat diarrhea, prevention (with insecticide-treated mosquito nets) and treatment of malaria, and treatment of pneumonia with antibiotics. Ongoing research is needed to help quantify the effect and the effectiveness of interventions in different settings.

Community-based approaches

Scale-up of integrated, community-based nutrition programs linked with health, water and sanitation, and other relevant interventions is a priority strategy that can bring measurable improvements in children's nutritional status, survival and development. Community support can include providing services such as counseling, support and communication on IYCN; screening for acute malnutrition and follow-up of malnourished children; deworming; and delivering vitamin A and micronutrient supplements. Synergizing nutrition-specific interventions with other early child development interventions at the community level is also important for holistically promoting early child development and reducing inequalities.

Communication for behavior and social change

Based on formative research on the barriers to and the facilitators of good nutrition, communication for behavior and social change can promote behavior change in communities, raise awareness about nutrition services and stimulate shifts in social norms in order to improve the enabling environment for good nutrition in communities.

Maintaining the focus on equity

Maintaining a focus on equity is particularly important, because stunting and other forms of undernutrition are concentrated among the most disadvantaged in society.

Undernutrition is inextricably linked with poverty. Equity-focused nutrition programming and other development strategies can effectively address the inequalities caused by poverty and the forms of exclusion that exist among groups and individuals.

For biological reasons, women and children are more vulnerable to nutritional deficiencies; special efforts are therefore needed to address the biological and social inequities that affect them. Women's low education levels, unequal social status and limited decision-making power can negatively influence the nutrition status of their children, as well as their own. Improving access to education and creating opportunities for both girls and boys, and their families, will confer many benefits in terms of nutritional status and child development.

Creating an enabling environment that targets the needs of vulnerable people is crucial. Since inequalities in nutritional status have a long-lasting, intergenerational impact on a country's physical, social and economic well-being, the response by communities and governments has implications for the nation's pursuit of equitable development.

The way forward

Over the past few years, national and global interest in nutrition has increased dramatically. There are a number of reasons for this new interest.

Recurrent food shortages, rising food prices and humanitarian crises in some regions have garnered global attention. The debate on climate change and the focus on building resilience in communities under stress have also focused attention on nutrition. At the other end of the spectrum, the rising numbers of people who struggle with overweight and obesity have become more glaring.

More persuasive evidence has become available on the harmful consequences of micronutrient deficiencies and the positive impact of exclusive breastfeeding and adequate complementary feeding for adult life and the next generation. At the same time, evidence has improved on the effectiveness of program approaches to treat conditions such as severe acute malnutrition using ready-to-use therapeutic foods and iron and folic acid deficiency using supplementation and wheat flour fortification – as well as on the feasibility of implementing these programs at scale.

Scientific knowledge and understanding have also improved regarding the linkages between stunting and rapid and disproportionate weight gain in early childhood. This has resulted in a shift in response. Previously the focus was on efforts to reduce the prevalence of underweight among children under the age of 5, an indicator of MDG 1. Now it is shifting towards prevention of stunting during the period from pregnancy up to 2 years of age.

The improved scientific evidence on the impact of interventions has enhanced advocacy to position nutrition as a sound investment for poverty reduction and social and economic development.

A unified international nutrition community has been using the Scaling Up Nutrition (SUN) Movement to successfully advocate for reduction of stunting, acute malnutrition and micronutrient deficiencies. This message has been heard and echoed by other initiatives and channels, including the Secretary-General's Zero Hunger Challenge, the 1,000 Days initiative and the Copenhagen Consensus 2012 Expert Panel's findings that malnourishment should be the top priority for policy-makers and philanthropists. The G8 has also included action to address stunting and other forms of undernutrition in its agenda.

By mid-2013, the SUN message had led 40 countries in Africa, Asia and Latin America to scale up their nutrition programs, supported by a wide range of organizations and, in many cases, by the donor community. This is probably the clearest indication of the growing interest in tackling stunting and other forms of undernutrition. It is crucial to maintain this momentum and to further increase the level of interest and motivation.

Nutrition-sensitive approaches

Nutrition-sensitive approaches involve other sectors in indirectly addressing the underlying causes of undernutrition. There is less evidence for the impact of nutrition-sensitive approaches than for direct nutrition-specific interventions, in part because they are hard to measure. However, policies and programming in agriculture, education, social protection and poverty reduction are important for realizing nutrition goals. Achieving nutrition-sensitive development requires multi-sectoral coordination and cooperation with many stakeholders, which has historically been challenging in nutrition. Agriculture and social protection programs are discussed in more detail below.

Agriculture

Recently, attention has increasingly been paid to improving synergies and linkages between agriculture and nutrition and health, in both the programmatic and the research communities.

The global agricultural system is currently producing enough food to feed the world, but access to adequate, affordable, nutritious food is more challenging. Improving dietary diversity by increasing production of nutritious foods is achievable, particularly in rural populations. It is done by producing nutrient-dense foods, such as fruits and vegetables, fish, livestock, milk and eggs; increasing the nutritional content of foods through crop biofortification and post-harvest fortification; improving storage and preservation of foods to cover 'lean' seasons; and educating people about nutrition and diet. In several settings these types of interventions have been shown to improve dietary patterns and intake of specific micronutrients, either directly or by increasing household income. However, the impact on stunting, wasting and micronutrient deficiencies is less clear.

More effort is needed to align the pursuit of food security with nutrition security and improved nutritional outcomes.

Social protection

Social protection involves policies and programs that protect people against vulnerability, mitigate the impacts of shocks, improve resilience and support people whose livelihoods are at risk. Safety nets are a type of social protection that provides or substitutes for income: Targeted cash transfers and food-access-based approaches are the two main categories of safety nets intended to avert starvation and reduce undernutrition among the most vulnerable populations. Food-based safety nets are designed to ensure livelihoods (such as public works employment paid in food), increase purchasing power (through food stamps, coupons or vouchers) and relieve deprivation (by providing food directly to households or individuals).

While social safety net programs operate in at least a dozen countries, evidence indicating that these programs have improved child nutritional status is still limited. A review of evaluations of conditional cash transfer programs showed an impact on stunting in two of five studies, the *Familias en Acción* program in Colombia and the *Oportunidades* program in Mexico. Of the three unconditional cash transfer programs, two (South African Child Support Grants and Ecuador's *Bono Solidario*) reduced stunting. More research and evidence is needed on the long-term outcomes of these programs and how they can be better targeted, how long they are needed and with what interventions. But social safety net programs may be one way to ensure more equitable nutrition-sensitive development if they are aligned with local and national needs and an understanding of capacity, resources and timeliness aspects in scaling up.

101

My personal view

Werner Schultink
Associate Director,
UNICEF

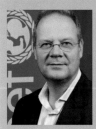

A number of common determinants are fundamental to successful implementation. These include the political commitment to reduce stunting and other forms of undernutrition; the design and implementation of comprehensive and effective national policy and programs based on sound situation analysis; the presence of trained and skilled community workers collaborating with communities; effective communication and advocacy; and multi-sectoral delivery of services.

Now that many countries are scaling up nutrition programs, it is important to ensure optimal use of resources and achieve results rapidly. If programs are not making the necessary progress, strategies need to be adapted quickly. This requires a monitoring system to assess whether bottlenecks impeding program effectiveness are effectively addressed and the collection of information in real time rather than reliance on large-scale household survey data, which are normally collected intermittently.

The evidence demonstrating the impact of stunting and other forms of undernutrition on survival, individual and national development, and long-term health is irrefutable.

As the world looks to the post-2015 development agenda, it is clear that prevention and treatment of undernutrition must be at its core. The evidence outlined in this chapter, the momentum around tackling the problem, the successes already achieved and the impact on equitable and sustainable poverty reduction show that improving child and maternal nutrition is both achievable and imperative for global progress.

Further reading

UNICEF. *Improving Child Nutrition: The achievable imperative for global progress. New York, NY, USA: UNICEF, 2013.*

Save the Children. Surviving the first day: State of the world's mothers 2013.

World Health Organization. Essential Nutrition Actions: Improving maternal, newborn, infant and young child nutrition. Geneva: WHO 2013.

2013 Lancet Series on Maternal and Child Nutrition.

World Health Organization. Global nutrition policy review: What does it take to scale up nutrition action? Geneva: WHO 2013.

Chapter Eight

Taming Volatile Food Prices: A Prerequisite for Improving Nutrition

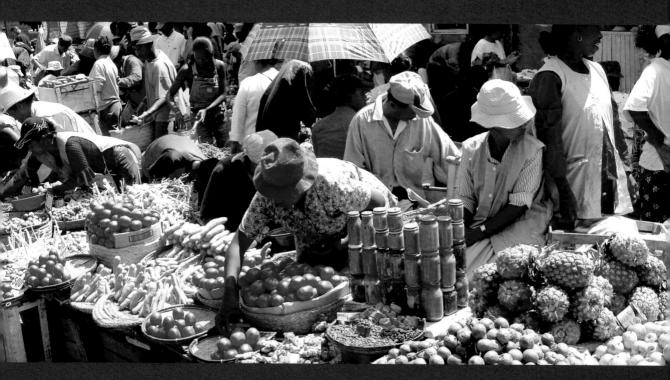

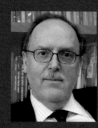

Joachim von Braun

Director of the Center for Development Research (ZEF)
Professor for Economic and Technological Change,
University of Bonn, Germany

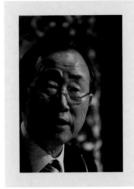

"We have the resources and the knowledge to end hunger. We know how to protect the poorest from the impact of rising prices. We know how to tame volatile prices. Every child, woman and man has a right to enough nutritious food for an active and healthy life. Let us act – now."

Ban Ki-moon, World Food Day Commemoration, 2011

Key messages

- Food prices today are not only set by supply and demand but also influenced by financial markets.

- Sudden price rises, or 'spikes', cause big problems for nutrition of the poor.

- Healthy diets need to be affordable, and that requires increased productivity in the food system to prevent high prices.

- Poor countries are hit worst as they cannot afford adjustment measures.

- The solution needs to be worked on globally, and the issue taken more seriously.

There are more than 800 million people seriously undernourished in the world today, and two billion suffering from hidden hunger. The price of food is a key factor in this situation.

Recent years have witnessed extreme fluctuations in the prices of food commodities. The basic cause is lack of agricultural productivity; additional factors include financial market volatility, political instability, and armed conflict. Others are scarcity of natural resources such as land and water, and rising energy prices.

The situation becomes even more complex when agricultural subsidies provided by governments in the West to their own farmers are considered – a factor that played an important role in the past – or when exports are restricted, which in recent years led to further scarcity and sudden price hikes in the global market. And it seems the countries giving out the subsidies are not without their problems either. In the US and Egypt, it has been argued that the artificially low prices can lead to unhealthy incentives for consumers. When energy-dense foods such as grains and sugar become cheaper, it is argued that these attract low-income families, leading to problems with overweight and obesity.

All of these factors and the price fluctuations that result have put pressure not just on individuals but on entire social groupings and, indeed, societies as a whole. Dramatic increases – or 'spikes' – in the cost of commodity foods have not only impoverished the diet and constrained the possibilities of many of the world's poorest and most vulnerable populations; they have in some instances actually led to food riots which have triggered major political and societal changes. The 'Arab Spring' that commenced on 18 December 2010 had complex causes, but food prices did play some role in triggering the violent change.

This chapter examines the various factors that influence food pricing, the repercussions experienced when price rises are deemed excessive, and solutions that could help alleviate the problem. Food price volatility is an issue that needs to be addressed on a global scale, rather than by individual countries only, for it is the poorer nations that suffer most in the wake of a food pricing crisis, as they are unable to fund the social and economic mitigation. Furthermore, not

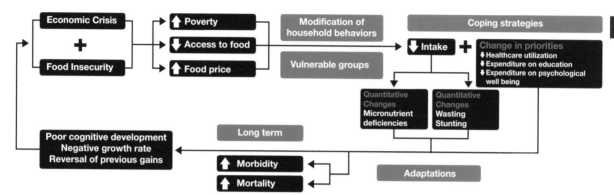

The vicious cycle of the economic crisis
Source: *Maternal and Young Child Nutrition Adversely Affected by External Shocks Such as Increasing Global Food Prices, Ian Darnton-Hill and Bruce Cogill, Journal of Nutrition 2010*

only do the sudden or short-term crises need to be addressed, but also the chronic situation that needs a coordinated and long-term response. One feature of that is the relative price increase of pulses, animal products and vegetables compared to calorie-dense foods, which leads to unhealthy diets of poor consumers, for instance in South Asia.

The effect of food price increases

Food prices around the globe are tracked by the Food Price Index, managed by the FAO (Food and Agricultural Organization). Strange as it may sound, the fact that food prices are either high or low in absolute terms is not the main destabilizing factor. The most serious problem occurs when a sudden change or 'spike' in prices occurs, for countries whose nutrition security is already compromised find it very hard to cope with these changes. Traditionally, such sudden price increases have been attributable to natural disasters such as droughts and floods, and to man-made disasters such as wars. Such occurrences limit the supply of food available. As supply dwindles but demand grows due to population and income growth, the result is inevitably higher prices for such produce.

If this is a phenomenon as old as money itself, there are also more recent factors that play a significant role in triggering food price spikes. One is the growing demand for high-end foods such as meat and dairy products on the part of the burgeoning middle classes of China and India. Another is the high price of oil in our oil-based global economy, which drives up the cost of every type of economic activity. A third was the global decline of food stocks in the last decade, for agricultural productivity growth had been declining worldwide for a number of years. Perhaps the most important, however, is the nature of the global commodities market.

During the past decade, there have been notable spikes in the period of 2007–8 and again in 2011. In certain countries, food prices were found to be three times as high in mid-2008 as the five-year average for that particular time of year. Prices rose again in mid-2010 because fears regarding droughts in Russia and parts of Asia affected stock levels.

The relationship between food production and pricing has a number of important dynamics:

1) When prices rise, the cost of acquiring food poses a growing problem. This is the most obvious effect. In order to prioritize the purchase of food within the framework of an unchanged budget, cuts have to be made elsewhere. On a household level, this can result in a general lowering of living standards, while governments may have to reduce funding for certain initiatives not related directly to the provision of food.

2) If the food in question becomes unobtainable on account of its increased price, the quality of the diet will deteriorate. Malnutrition leads to short-term health problems, but it also lays the foundation for long-term problems such as stunting and an increased predisposition to non-communicable diseases such as cardiovascular disease and type 2 diabetes. The undernutrition rate of the under-fives also rises, and the increased prevalence of these conditions has a lasting negative influence not only on the individuals affected but also upon the entire societies of which they form a part.

3) Changes in the price of food can also impact the macro-economy and labor markets, causing wages to rise or fall concomitantly. The worst-case scenario is when a drop in job opportunities is accompanied by a rise in food prices, as was the case in parts of the Arab region in recent years.

4) Difficulties caused by rising food prices will prompt a reaction from government. One response is to widen the social safety net, putting emergency schemes in place for the most economically vulnerable, but poor countries lack the resources for that and the effectiveness and coverage of such measures is often limited. Another response is to tax or otherwise legislate for the import or export of food, which has adverse effects for reliable trade flows.

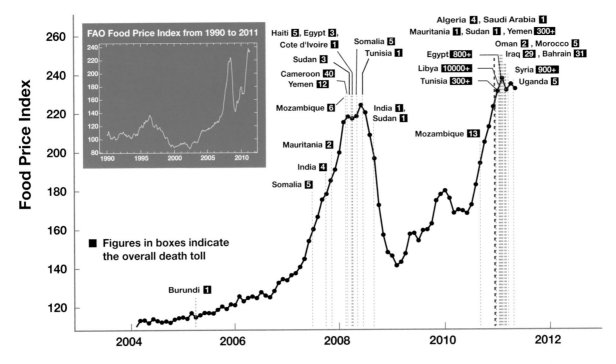

Time dependence of FAO Food Price Index from January 2004 to May 2011. Red dashed vertical lines correspond to beginning dates of "food riots" and protests associated with the major recent unrest in North Africa and the Middle East. The overall death toll is reported in parentheses. The blue vertical line indicates the date, December 13, 2010, on which we submitted a report to the U.S. government, warning of the link between food prices, social unrest and political instability. Inset shows FAO Food Price Index from 1990 to 2011. From The Food Crises and Political Instability in North Africa and the Middle East, Marco Lagi, Karla Z. Bertrand and Yaneer Bar-Yam, New England Complex Systems Institute, Cambridge, US

Double blow to the poor

In the wake of a food pricing crisis, it is the poor that suffer most. In fact, poor people spend an estimated 50–70 percent of their wages on food, and are unable to adapt to price rises, with wages for unskilled labor also unlikely to rise. The result is that households tend to limit their food consumption, eat less balanced diets, and spend less on goods and services. A vicious cycle of nutritional and economic deprivation is thus initiated.

The current economic climate can pose further problems, with falling wages and unemployment widespread in many parts of the world. Some three quarters of the world's poor live in rural areas. They are therefore more exposed to the impact of commodity price increases occurring in the global economy. China and India both attempted after 2008–9 to combat the problem of food price spikes by shielding themselves from the international market, and keeping all their national produce for domestic use. While successful in the short term, protectionist measures of this kind can negatively affect a country's global trading position, and therefore its wealth, in the longer term.

Food prices and the Arab Spring

While there were other contributing factors to the recent Arab Spring uprisings, food prices and the inability of governments to react to their increase were definitely part of it. The Middle East and North Africa are more dependent on imported food than other regions, and in 2007–8 when global food prices spiked, countries like Egypt were faced with rises in local food prices of 37 percent. With unemployment in the country rising also, people depended on the government to supply subsidies, but it was widely felt that not enough was being done. Food inflation in Egypt continued to rise, and was 18.9 percent when President Mubarak gave up his seat.

Other countries experienced difficulties, with Bahrain, Yemen, Jordan and Morocco all staging food demonstrations during 2008. Many governments offered subsidies, but as in the case of Egypt, these were deemed low quality and not enough. In Egypt and Yemen, over 40 percent of the population live below the poverty line and suffer malnutrition, while 30 percent of Egyptian adults and 35 percent of Jordanians are obese. According to the Gallup World Poll, between half and three quarters of the Arab population say they are unhappy with their government's poverty reduction efforts. "The food-price spike was the final nail in the coffin for regimes that were failing to deliver on their side of the social contract," Jane Harrigan of London's School of Oriental and African Studies told the Economist.

Sources: http://www.economist.com/node/21550328, http://www.guardian. co.uk/lifeandstyle/2011/jul/17/bread-food-arab-spring

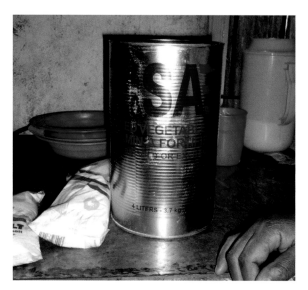

Can containing fortified vegetable oil
Source: Mike Bloem Photography

How are food prices set?

Food pricing today is no longer set by the straightforward dynamics of supply and demand only. A report published by the United Nations Conference on Trade and Development in 2000 and entitled *Commodity Exchanges in a Globalized Economy* provides an introduction to the topic.

"Modern commodity exchanges date back to the trading of rice futures in the 17th century in Osaka, Japan, although the principles that underpin commodity futures trading and the function of commodity markets are still older. The first recorded account of derivative contracts can be traced to the ancient Greek philosopher Thales of Miletus in Greece, who, during the winter, negotiated what were essentially called options on oil presses for the spring olive harvest. The Spanish dramatist Lope de Vega reported that in the 17th century options and futures were traded on the Amsterdam Bourse [Stock Exchange] soon after it was opened."

It continues:

"Futures' trading is a natural application to the problems of maintaining a year-round supply of seasonal products like agricultural crops. Exchanging traded futures and options provides several economic benefits, including the ability to shift or otherwise manage the price risk of market or tangible positions. With the liberalization of agricultural trade in many countries, and the withdrawal of government support to agricultural producers, there is a new need for price discovery and even physical trading mechanisms, a need that can often be met by commodity exchanges. Hence, the rapid creation of new commodity exchanges."

Commodity exchanges are places where commodities and derivatives are traded. This generally covers agricultural produce and other raw materials (e.g. wheat, sugar and maize) and contracts based on them. These contracts may be the basis for a range of sophisticated financial products including, for instance, futures, interest rates and swaps. Futures are future contracts on a crop that has not yet been harvested. They set the sale price in advance for both the producer (the farmer) and the purchaser (e.g. a food processor). Both producer and purchaser are thereby protected from potential price fluctuations at the moment of sale. The price of grain crops – especially of wheat, corn and soy – is set in this manner. Food commodities are assets worth investing in, and are treated in the same way as stocks or bonds. Investors will buy a package of food commodities through a hedge fund, and ask them to be traded at a time that is financially opportune.

Milk prices, by contrast, are derived from feed prices, while rice prices are set at a national level, as rice is such an important staple food in so many parts of the world.

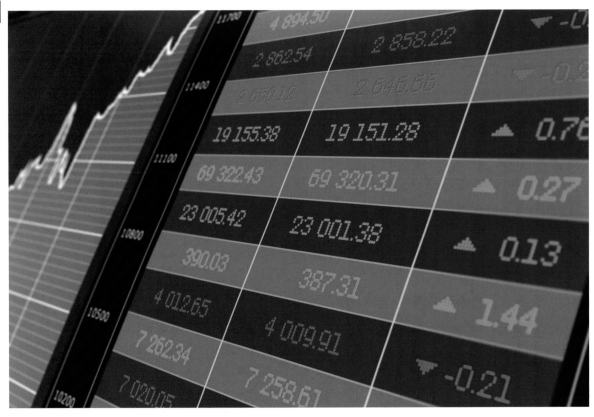

Case study

Case study: Guatemala

A study conducted in Guatemala in 2008 revealed that the price of a diet based on a corn tortilla, vegetable oil, vegetables and beans – containing key recommended micronutrients – is twice the cost of a less nutritious diet based only a tortilla and oil. The cost of the diet for one person with beans and vegetables is also around a third of the total household income of a family living on $1 a day.

If a person were to eat the diet based only on the tortilla and oil, they would receive no vitamin A and C, and very low levels of other essential nutrients. This will put them at risk in terms of health problems and illnesses, some of which can be long term.

Source: Erick Boy, IFPRI, based on Guatemala City market prices in November 2008; and data from FAO/WHO 2002

Abstract

A food crisis occurs when rates of hunger and malnutrition rise sharply at local, national, or global levels. This definition distinguishes a food crisis from chronic hunger, although food crises are far more likely among populations already suffering from prolonged hunger and malnutrition. A food crisis is usually set off by a shock to either supply or demand for food and often involves a sudden spike in food prices. It is important to remember that in a market economy, food prices measure the scarcity of food, not its value in any nutritional sense. Except in rare circumstances, the straightforward way to prevent a food crisis is to have rapidly rising labor productivity through economic growth and keep food prices stable while maintaining access by the poor. The formula is easier to state than to implement, especially on a global scale, but it is good to have both the objective, reducing short-run spikes in hunger, and the deep mechanisms, pro-poor economic growth and stable food prices, clearly in mind. A coherent food policy seeks to use these mechanisms, and others, to achieve a sustained reduction in chronic hunger over the long run while preventing spikes in hunger in the short run.

Source: J. Nutr. 140: 224S–228S, 2010.

It is ironic that the prices of many food commodities are today partly decided by financial markets that have nothing to do with the process of producing food by agriculture or with the procedure for distributing it physically within an economy. Cuts in food prices can have a drastic effect on the farmers who actually grow the food. At the same time, sharp increases in food prices can threaten the well-being of the poorest sections of society, who have no means to increase their income in response to the rising cost of food.

Links between the food and financial crises

Looking at the dates where the worst spikes in rising food prices occurred recently, in 2007–8 and 2011, one could easily assume that a direct connection must exist between the rise of food commodity prices and the more widespread global economic crisis which occurred during the same period. The relationship is somewhat more complex, however.

Before the global recession, the consumption of agricultural products increased in line with income and population figures, rising energy prices and subsidized biofuel production. Pressure was placed on production, however, by natural resource constraints, underinvestment in rural infrastructure and agricultural science, and weather disruptions.

The much wider financial crisis of 2008, which started in the USA and resulted in the collapse of the housing and financial markets in many parts of the world, led to increased speculation surrounding agricultural commodities, introducing volatility and making prices rise further.

Global Food: Waste Not, Want Not

Feeding the 9 Billion: The Tragedy of Waste

By 2075, the United Nations' predicts human numbers will peak at about 9.5 billion people – an extra 3 billion mouths to feed. Substantial changes are anticipated in the wealth, calorific intake and dietary preferences of people in developing countries. However 30–50% (or 1.2–2 billion tons) of all food produced never reaches a human stomach.

Developing nations

In less-developed countries, wastage occurs primarily at the farmer-producer end of the supply chain due to inefficient harvesting, inadequate local transportation and poor infrastructure. As development increases, the problem generally moves further up the supply chain with regional and national infrastructure deficiencies having the largest impact.

Developed nations

In fully developed countries such as the UK, a larger proportion of the food produced reaches markets and consumers. However produce is often wasted through retail and customer behavior.

Major supermarkets often reject crops because they do not meet exacting marketing standards. Up to 30% of the UK's vegetable crop is never harvested as a result of such practices. Globally, retailers generate 1.6 million tons of food waste annually in this way.

Sales promotions encourage customers to purchase excessive quantities, which generates wastage of perishable foodstuffs. Between 30% and 50% of food bought in developed countries is thrown away.

Better use of our finite resources

Wasting food is a waste of land, water and energy. Tackling of food waste involves addressing key resource issues:

Effective land usage

Over the last five decades, improved farming techniques and 12% expansion of farmed land have increased crop production. Further expansion of crop land would impact on the world's natural ecosystems. Per capita calorific intake from meat consumption is set to rise 40% by mid-century, and meat products require significantly more resources and land to produce. Considerable tensions are likely to emerge, as the need for food competes with demands for ecosystem preservation and biomass production as a renewable energy source.

Water usage

Over the past century, fresh water withdrawal for human use has increased at more than double the rate of population growth. The demand for water in food production could reach 10–13 trillion m^3 annually by mid-century. This is 2.5 to 3.5 times greater than the total human use of fresh water today.

About 40% of the world's food supply is currently derived from irrigated land. However, water used in irrigation is often sourced unsustainably, and we continue to use wasteful systems. While drip or trickle irrigation methods are more expensive to install, they can be 33% more efficient and carry fertilizers directly to the root.

In the production of foods besides crops, especially in meat production, there are large additional uses of water. More effective procedures, and recycling and purification of water will be needed to reduce wastage.

Energy usage

An average of 7–10 calories of input is required in the production of one calorie of food. This varies dramatically depending on crop, from three calories for plant crops to 35 calories for beef.

High productivity in agricultural crops requires appropriate fertilizer use. In the modern industrialized agricultural process the making and application of agrochemicals such as fertilizers and pesticides represents the single biggest energy component. Wheat production takes 50% of its energy input from these two items alone. Fertilizer manufacturing consumes 3–5% of the world's annual natural gas supply. With production anticipated to increase by 25% between now and 2030, sustainable energy sourcing will become an increasingly major issue.

Source: Aggidis G, Arbon I, Brown, C et al, Global Food – Waste Not, Want Not, The Institution of Mechanical Engineers, January 2013

The long-term health risks of rising food prices

Micronutrient deficiencies can lead to a wide number health problems, including impaired cognitive development, lower resistance to disease, and increased risks during childbirth for both mothers and children.

It is essential that governments do not undervalue or underestimate the long-term effects to the population caused by rising food prices. There is a short-term effect that food will be hard for the population to budget for and that bad diets may be eaten, with a serious risk of long-terms problems arising from this situation. Careful monitoring and assistance should be provided by governments when a food pricing crisis is under way, and also for a suitable length of time afterwards.

This would require funds set aside by the government to ensure its recovery from the crisis and also that of the population. Data will need to be collected, and assessed, in addition to the right aid and support, and potentially supplementary foods provided, to limit any long-term effects.

Source: Overcoming the World Food and Agriculture Crisis through Policy Change, Institutional Innovation, and Science, Joachim von Braun, TAAS Lecture. New Delhi, March 6, 2009. http://www.taas.in/documents/fdl4_jvbraun.pdf

How does climate change affect food prices?

Food production is very sensitive to climate change, and a small crop yield as the result of drought, too much rainfall, or extremes like flooding or storms, can push prices up. The effect of global warming is resulting in greater weather extremes than ever before, with bigger impacts on food production, felt around the world. In Russia in summer 2012, a heat wave destroyed around a third of its crop yield, while in the US, the worst drought experienced by the country in 50 years destroyed almost half the corn crop and a third of the soya bean crop.

Richard Tiffin, director for the Centre of Food Security at the University of Reading in the UK said:

"It should be a major warning that climate change is increasingly having a global impact on the food supply. If the problems in Russia and the US were combined with a failure of the Indian monsoon, we could see a major global food crisis that would have an enormous impact on food prices and badly affect poor people around the world."

A recent study by Stanford University suggests that the global production of maize and wheat since 1980 would have been 5% higher if not for climate change. Increases in carbon dioxide in the atmosphere is actually said to be beneficial to the production of certain crops, such as rice, soybean and wheat, but climate change will affect the length and quality of the growing season, and the overall effect of climate change on world agricultural production is clearly negative.

Sources: http://www.guardian.co.uk/environment/damian-carrington-blog/2012/oct/10/food-price-rise-uk-crop-harvest http://www.guardian.co.uk/environment/2012/sep/19/climate-change-affect-food-production

What happens next?

While challenges regarding food reserves and pricing have populated the headlines in recent years, many experts believe that more risks are on the way.

Food consumption is said to have exceeded growth for six of the past 11 years, with yields of most crops, excluding rice, falling. According to the FAO, food prices rose 1.4 percent in September and 6 percent in July.

The key to solving the global food crisis and preventing prices from escalating further lies at a global level. It is important that all countries come together and accept shared responsibility. The risks regarding food price spikes and their repercussions were known many years before the dangerous increases occurred, but governments failed to give them sufficient credence. For example, only twice in the past 10 years has food been listed in the top five factors for the Global Risk Report.

A potential solution to rising food prices lies in the following areas:

1. Promote sustainable intensification of agriculture growth

Governments should increase their investments in R&D, rural infrastructure, rural institutions, and information monitoring and sharing of scientific insight. Smallholders need improved access to affordable finance. Investments in agriculture would increase output, helping countries to emerge from poverty.

2. Reduce market volatility

A lack of information can lead to market inefficiencies and reduce the extent of mutually beneficial exchanges. Investors need more transparency about market information and stocks. Appropriate regulation of commodity exchanges is called for.

3. Expand social protection and child nutrition action

Preventative actions are needed to address both short-term and long-term issues. This could include conditional cash transfers, pension systems and employment programs, while children could benefit from supplementary feeding in the first two years, school feeding, and increased food education.

In addition to this framework, borders must remain open, and sharing scarcity through trade should not be reduced. Export restrictions should be avoided, as this leads to a smaller import/export market, which keeps prices high. Food aid should be allowed to flow freely between countries. The solution to the problem of food price spikes lies in our hands, but it will take a global effort of concentrated willpower to make those hands work effectively together.

My personal view

Joachim von Braun
Director of the Center for Development Research (ZEF)
Professor for Economic and Technological Change,
University of Bonn, Germany

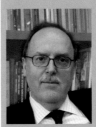

Food security – the availability of and access to sufficient and healthy foods and good nutrition – is central to the well-being of nations and people. Food insecurity has increased in the context of the inter-linked food price and economic crises of 2007–08 and again in 2010–11. The food price crisis is mainly a consequence of neglected investment in agriculture in many developing countries, inappropriate agriculture energy subsidization policies in industrialized countries, and then triggered by adverse weather events and exacerbated further by export restrictions. The consequences are volatile and spiking food prices that undermine food and nutrition security of the poor. A comprehensive assessment of the costs of price volatility is called for; including human costs, adverse investment effects, macro-economic and fiscal effects, and market distortions such as speculation. Empirical analysis of the inter-linkages of food, energy and financial markets suggests that food security policy needs to go beyond traditional mitigation of demand- and supply-side shocks. And a comprehensive portfolio of policy actions for prevention of price spikes is proposed here, including better regulation of commodity exchanges and innovative food reserves policies.

Further reading

IFPRI website: www. foodsecurityportal.org

Food and Agriculture Organization. The State of Food Insecurity in the World. Rome: FAO 2012.

von Braun J. Increasing and More Volatile Food Prices and the Consumer. In: The Oxford Handbook of the Economics of Food Consumption and Policy, 2012. DOI:10.1093/ oxfordhb/9780199569441.013.0025

Chapter Nine

Making Nutrition Good Politics: The Power of Governance

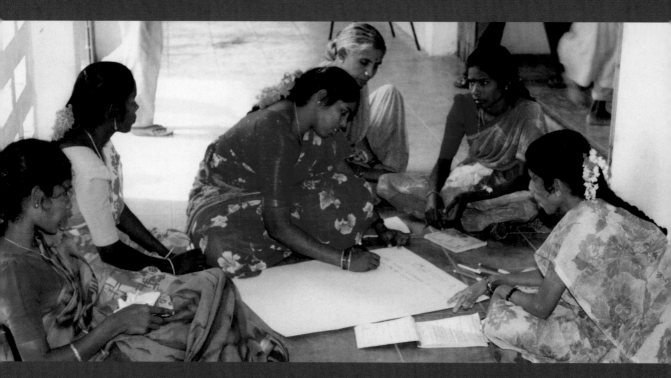

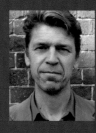

Stuart Gillespie
Senior Research Fellow, Poverty, Health and Nutrition Division, International Food Policy
Researc Institute (IFPRI)
CEO of the Transform Nutrition Research Program Consortium
Currently based in Brighton, UK

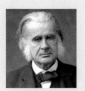

"There is no sea more dangerous than the ocean of practical politics – none in which there is more need of good pilots and of a single, unfaltering purpose when the waves rise high."

Thomas Henry Huxley – *physiologist, anatomist, anthropologist and early champion of Darwin's Theory of Evolution, (1825–1895)*

Key messages

- Undernutrition has certain features which necessitate a strong focus on governance.

- Progress in reducing undernutrition cannot be sustained where governance systems are weak or absent.

- As governance relates to power, capacity, commitment, accountability and responsiveness, it is crucially important for *all* levels of action, not just the policy level.

- Strong leadership – in the form of ambassadors championing the political cause, as well as more midlevel, lateral leadership to facilitate intersectoral action- is fundamental to success.

- Governance can be measured and monitored using innovative new tools and indices, with the results used to name, shame and praise.

What is good governance, and why is it needed for nutrition security?

The concept of governance has many definitions. Governance can be defined with regard to institutional structures, relationships between actors and/or organizations, decision-making processes, and incentives. It involves the capacity to act, the power to act and the commitment to act. It requires accountability, responsiveness and transparency. Essentially, good governance refers to the effective, efficient, accountable exercise of public authority for the provision of a public good.

The challenge of undernutrition has several features which require strong systems of governance to successfully address it.

First, the nature of the problem itself. Undernutrition is neglected because it is invisible, it is not infectious (unlike HIV, for example), it requires several actions to be undertaken by many actors in several unconnected sectors, and at different levels, it is difficult to measure success and to attribute impact to any one decision or action (unlike for example vaccinating a child against a disease), and the benefits of improving nutrition often take longer than a politician's time in office to fully manifest themselves. These unique features generate a lack of commitment, accountability and responsiveness to act, which – linked with the major challenge of limited leadership, strategic and operational capacity – all combine to fuel the political economy of undernutrition reduction.

The **second** fundamental rationale for a strong focus on governance is the type of action that is needed to ensure nutrition security.

Globally the challenge of overweight and obesity is growing but accelerating the reduction of undernutrition remains the major challenge in many countries. In these situations, ensuring nutrition security requires action on three broad fronts.

First, there's a need to enhance and expand the quality and coverage of *nutrition-specific* interventions. Second, maximizing the *nutrition-sensitivity* of more "indirect" interventions, such as agriculture, social protection, water and sanitation etc., And third, there is a need to cultivate and sustain enabling political and policy environments for nutrition. This third level – which largely relates to global and national governance – has been relatively neglected to date.

At this third level, the challenge is to understand how high-level political momentum can drive action to reduce undernutrition, and what needs to happen to turn this momentum into results on the ground. How to ensure that high-quality, well-resourced direct (nutrition-specific) interventions are available to those who need them, and indirect (nutrition-sensitive) actions (e.g. agriculture, social protection, water and sanitation) are re-oriented to support nutrition goals? These three levels of complementary action correspond broadly to the three levels of causes of undernutrition – immediate (individual) level, underlying (household, community) level and basic (national and global) levels.

But governance is not only an issue for policy and politicians. It is a key cross-cutting issue at all three levels of action described above. This is because direct interventions can fail to scale because of weak incentives, institutions and infrastructure, indirect interventions are often underleveraged for nutrition because of commitment and coordination failures, and the environment for nutrition is more often disabling due to the invisibility of undernutrition and weak leadership from the state and civil society.

The need for good governance to ensure nutrition security is thus incontestable. Sustained progress is simply not possible where governance systems are weak or absent.

Why is it so important now?

Yet the focus on governance has only emerged in recent years as two types of gaps or disconnects have emerged.

First, the disconnect between the strong evidence of the damage caused by malnutrition, on the one hand, and the relative inertia with regard to action, on the other. So much more is now known about the drivers of undernutrition and the serious and enduring consequences of undernutrition, the benefits of acting to reduce undernutrition, and the costs of inaction and/or poorly designed and implemented responses.

Second, the disconnect between sustained economic growth of several high-burden countries and their failure to make significant inroads in addressing undernutrition. This has been seen most dramatically in South Asia, though there are now signs of positive change in some countries (such as Nepal, and Bangladesh – see case study). As their nations grow economically, governments need to decide how important it is that their children grow. They may have the power and capacity (including financial resources) to act, but often they don't act (or not at the scale required) because they lack commitment.

Commitment has been likened to a political *will* to act – and this does not fall from the sky, it needs to be created. As James Grant, the former Executive Director of UNICEF said:

"Each of the great social achievements of recent decades has come about not because of government proclamations, but because people organized, made demands, and made it good politics for governments to respond. It is the political will of the people that makes and sustains the political will of governments."

This then throws the spotlight on accountability and responsiveness of political systems, how power is distributed, and how equitable societies and political systems are. Are governments held accountable for their actions or their failure to act? Are they *responsive* to changing situations, especially in context of humanitarian crises.

Politics and policy processes are now firmly embedded in the agenda of both research and action. No longer is the political economy of nutrition viewed as an impenetrable "black box". Nutrition advocates or champions, adept at navigating and shaping policy arenas, are emerging. More policy research is being done on these issues – often with multidisciplinary teams – to shine a light on success or failure and what drives it. We know a lot more now about the pathways and dynamics of change, the key levers and catalysts, and what drives success or failure (see "further reading").

Proportions of countries reporting the content of policies, by WHO region

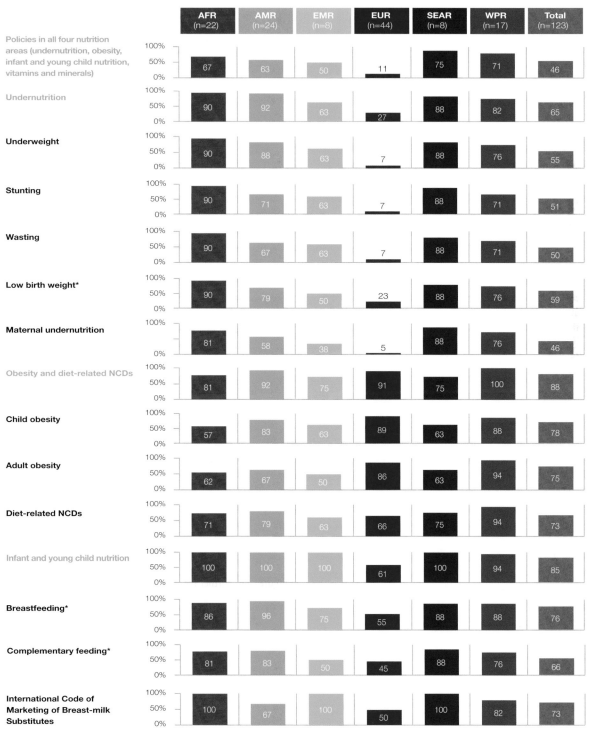

	AFR (n=22)	AMR (n=24)	EMR (n=8)	EUR (n=44)	SEAR (n=8)	WPR (n=17)	Total (n=123)
Policies in all four nutrition areas (undernutrition, obesity, infant and young child nutrition, vitamins and minerals)	67	63	50	11	75	71	46
Undernutrition	90	92	63	27	88	82	65
Underweight	90	88	63	7	88	76	55
Stunting	90	71	63	7	88	71	51
Wasting	90	67	63	7	88	71	50
Low birth weight*	90	79	50	23	88	76	59
Maternal undernutrition	81	58	38	5	88	76	46
Obesity and diet-related NCDs	81	92	75	91	75	100	88
Child obesity	57	83	63	89	63	88	78
Adult obesity	62	67	50	86	63	94	75
Diet-related NCDs	71	79	63	66	75	94	73
Infant and young child nutrition	100	100	100	61	100	94	85
Breastfeeding*	86	96	75	55	88	88	76
Complementary feeding*	81	83	50	45	88	76	66
International Code of Marketing of Breast-milk Substitutes	100	67	100	50	100	82	73

Source: WHO's Global nutrition policy review

115

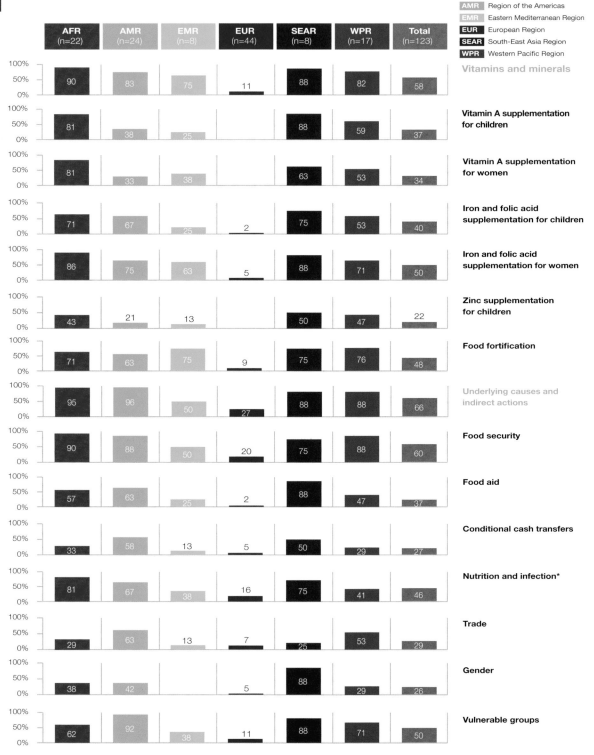

AFR   African Region
AMR   Region of the Americas
EMR   Eastern Mediterranean Region
EUR   European Region
SEAR   South-East Asia Region
WPR   Western Pacific Region

Vitamins and minerals

Vitamin A supplementation for children

Vitamin A supplementation for women

Iron and folic acid supplementation for children

Iron and folic acid supplementation for women

Zinc supplementation for children

Food fortification

Underlying causes and indirect actions

Food security

Food aid

Conditional cash transfers

Nutrition and infection*

Trade

Gender

Vulnerable groups

Source: WHO's Global nutrition policy review

Age-standardized prevalence of overweight and obesity in adults 20+ years of age by WHO region. 2008

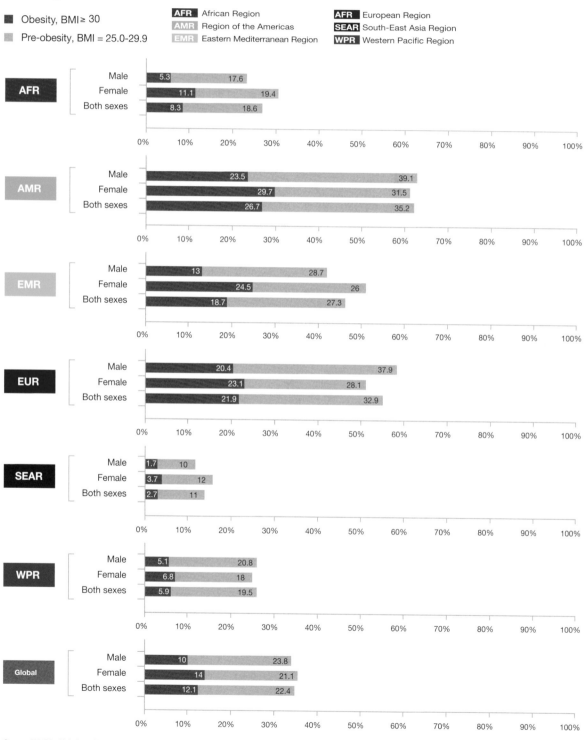

- ■ Obesity, BMI ≥ 30
- ▨ Pre-obesity, BMI = 25.0-29.9

AFR	African Region
AMR	Region of the Americas
EMR	Eastern Mediterranean Region

AFR	European Region
SEAR	South-East Asia Region
WPR	Western Pacific Region

Source: WHO's Global nutrition policy review

117 Policies, coordination mechanisms and stakeholders, interventions and surveillance in countries with high and low levels of stunting. Data are presented as the percentage of total number of countries in each group.

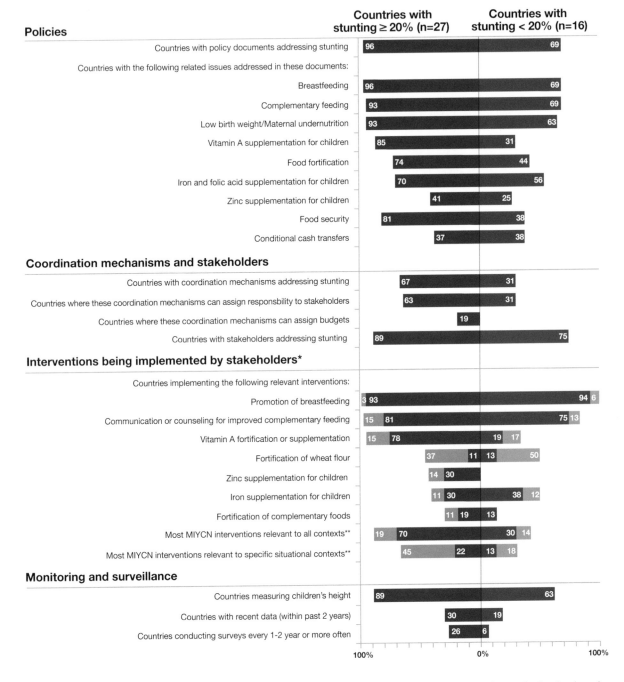

Note: * For interventions, the darker area indicates implementation at national scale, the lighter area indicates implementation at subnational scale, and the full bar implementation at any scale (national or subnational). ** This refers to a majority of maternal, infant and young child nutrition (MIYCN) interventions relevant to please all contexts or in specific situational contexts as identified by Bhutta et al. (2008) and listed in Table 4.

What are the core drivers and ingredients of good governance?

At the time of the 2008 Lancet Nutrition Series, the governance of the international nutrition system was said to have been fragmented and dysfunctional. Since then, a process of reforming UN institutional architecture has been underway, and the Scaling Up Nutrition (SUN) Movement has emerged with a core focus on galvanizing national and country-led action (see box).

The global architecture is now characterized by an array of governments, NGOs, international and regional organizations, donors, foundations, research organizations, academia and private foundations and companies. Compared to five years ago, there is much more coherence and complementarity in the way these different actors and organizations interact.

But the SUN Movement will ultimately only realize its true potential through its application in each country. This will require the maintenance of support and consensus amongst all SUN stakeholders, and strong country-level ownership.

Strong leadership – in the form of ambassadors championing the political cause, as well as more mid-level, lateral leadership to facilitate intersectoral action – is fundamental to success.

In terms of institutional arrangements, nutrition is an issue that needs an executive body, ideally linked to the Prime Minister's office, and a coordinating body that ensures horizontal (cross-sectoral) and vertical (national to district) coherence in action.

These two bodies need to ensure accountability and responsiveness through regular collection and management of key data on nutrition trends and changing drivers, ensuring the quality and appropriate scale-up of direct nutrition interventions (targeted to the 1,000-day window of opportunity), maximizing the nutrition-sensitivity of wider development programs (especially agriculture and social protection), and mobilizing and managing capacity and financing to sustain all these efforts.

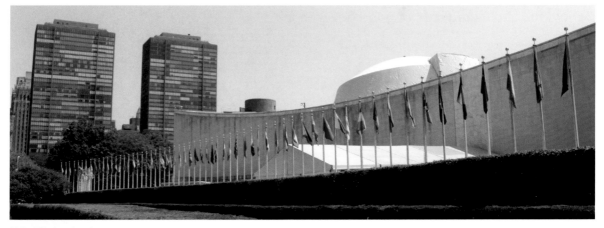

United Nations headquarters
Source: http://www.panoramio.com

How is governance measured and monitored?

Governance is key for all stages in the policy process – from agenda-setting, to policy formulation, program planning, implementation, monitoring and evaluation. It is fundamental for creating and sustaining commitment but also crucially for *converting* such commitment into real impact on the ground. Different challenges emerge at this point. The quality, intensity, and equity of implementation may not be as easily tracked as the existence of a plan or a legal framework, as shown by a landscape analysis. Understanding whether and how well policies are actually implemented and legal instruments are

enforced will require different measures and different perspectives, including importantly those of nutritionally vulnerable populations themselves.

In 2012, WHO introduced a comprehensive "'Landscape Analysis" mapping tool in order to assess nutrition governance in different countries. If a country has most or all of the following indicators in place, they could be described as having 'strong' nutrition governance, and good readiness to accelerate action in nutrition: political commitment and awareness of nutrition, focused policies and regulation at a central level, with supporting plans and protocols at subnational level, resource mobilization at central level and budget provision at subnational level, coordination of nutrition activities at all levels, involvement of partners, support to districts and facilities, trained staff with appropriate skills at all levels, capacity and motivation of staff, quality of services and follow up, management, information systems and supplies in place, and community engagement strategies.

The SUN Movement has a simple four indicator system to track country-level progress, including existence of a multi-stakeholder platform, coherent legal and political framework, alignment of policies and programs around a common results framework, and mobilization and tracking of financial resources.

Innovative tools are increasingly available to stimulate and build commitment and accountability. For governments and donors, for example, a Nutrition Commitment Index has been developed by the Institute of Development Studies for cross-country and country-specific comparisons over time.

This measures political commitment to tackle undernutrition in 45 developing countries by focusing on a series of policy, legal and spending indicators. The first analysis in early 2013 generated some interesting results – for example, some of the poorest developing countries are showing the greatest political commitment to tackling undernutrition, e.g., Malawi and Madagascar, while economic powerhouses such as India and Nigeria are failing some of their most vulnerable citizens. The index not only shows that low wealth is no barrier to committed action, it also highlights that sustained economic growth does not guarantee that governments will prioritize undernutrition reduction. This may help explain why many countries in sub-Saharan Africa and South Asia remain blighted by high levels of hunger and undernutrition. In naming, shaming and praising, such tools can be very powerful.

This is quite possible at more decentralized levels too – ICT-based monitoring systems, social accountability mechanisms, and community-based tools such as community scorecards, have all been shown to promote accountability and to improve the provision of direct public services.

Definitions and ingredients of good governance

In possibly the first statement defining "governance", in 1999, the World Bank defines national governance as:

"the traditions and institutions by which authority in a country is exercised. This includes the process by which governments are selected, monitored and replaced, the capacity of the government to effectively formulate and implement sound policies, and the respect of citizens and the state for the institutions that govern economic and social interactions among them.

(**Source**: *Kaufmann, D. and Kraay, A. (2008) Governance Indicators: Where are We, Where Should We Be Going? The World Bank Research Observer 23 91), 1–30.)*

"Governance is....the exercise of economic, political, and administrative authority to manage a country's affairs at all levels. It comprises mechanisms, processes, and institutions through which citizens and groups articulate their interests, exercise their legal rights, meet their obligations, and mediate their differences."

(**Source**: *Governance for Sustainable Human Development: A United Nations Development Program Policy Document, 14 April 2005)*

"Good governance refers to governing systems which are capable, responsible, inclusive and transparent. All countries, developed and developing, need to work continuously towards better governance."

(**Source**: *Helen Clark, Administrator of the UNDP. Fourth United Nations conference on the Least Developed Countries High Level Interactive Thematic Debate on Good Governance at All Levels, Istanbul, 11 May 2011)*

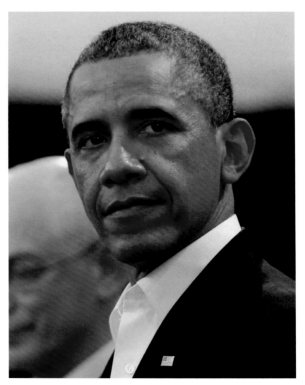

President Obama at the G8 Summit At Lough Erne
Source: WPA Pool (GETTY)

Hunger and Nutrition Commitment Index (HANCI) Scores

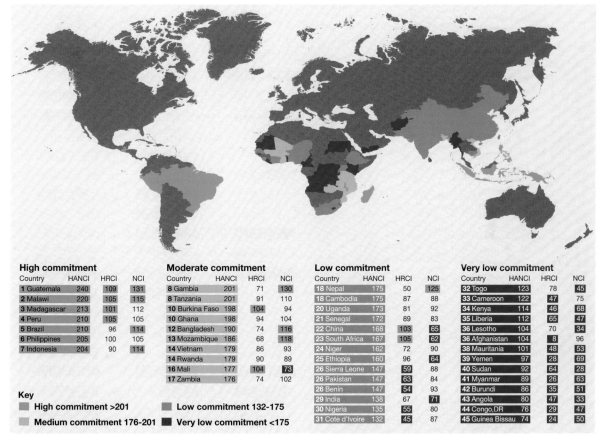

High commitment

Country	HANCI	HRCI	NCI
1 Guatemala	240	109	131
2 Malawi	220	105	115
3 Madagascar	213	101	112
4 Peru	210	105	105
5 Brazil	210	96	114
6 Philippines	205	100	105
7 Indonesia	204	90	114

Moderate commitment

Country	HANCI	HRCI	NCI
8 Gambia	201	71	130
8 Tanzania	201	91	110
10 Burkina Faso	198	104	94
10 Ghana	198	94	104
12 Bangladesh	190	74	116
13 Mozambique	186	68	118
14 Vietnam	179	86	93
14 Rwanda	179	90	89
16 Mali	177	104	73
17 Zambia	176	74	102

Low commitment

Country	HANCI	HRCI	NCI
18 Nepal	175	50	125
18 Cambodia	175	87	88
20 Uganda	173	81	92
21 Senegal	172	89	83
22 China	168	103	65
23 South Africa	167	105	62
24 Niger	162	72	90
25 Ethiopia	160	96	64
26 Sierra Leone	147	59	88
26 Pakistan	147	63	84
26 Benin	147	54	93
29 India	138	67	71
30 Nigeria	135	55	80
31 Cote d'Ivoire	132	45	87

Very low commitment

Country	HANCI	HRCI	NCI
32 Togo	123	78	45
33 Cameroon	122	47	75
34 Kenya	114	46	68
35 Liberia	112	65	47
36 Lesotho	104	70	34
36 Afghanistan	104	8	96
38 Mauritania	101	48	53
39 Yemen	97	28	69
40 Sudan	92	64	28
41 Myanmar	89	26	63
42 Burundi	86	35	51
43 Angola	80	47	33
44 Congo,DR	76	29	47
45 Guinea Bissau	74	24	50

Key

- High commitment >201
- Medium commitment 176-201
- Low commitment 132-175
- Very low commitment <175

Hunger Reduction Commitment Index (HRCI) Scores

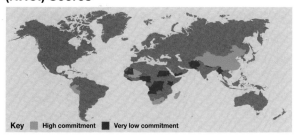

Key High commitment Very low commitment

Nutrition Commitment Index (NCI) Scores

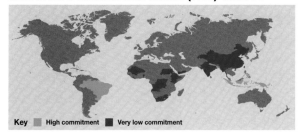

Key High commitment Very low commitment

The structure of the HANCI

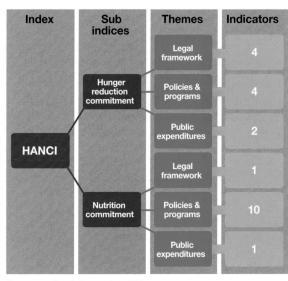

Index	Sub indices	Themes	Indicators
	Hunger reduction commitment	Legal framework	4
		Policies & programs	4
		Public expenditures	2
HANCI	Nutrition commitment	Legal framework	1
		Policies & programs	10
		Public expenditures	1

Source: www.hancindex.org, June 2013

121

Landscape Analysis:

Country progress in reaching MDG1 nutrition target		PRSP*	UNDAF**	Nutrition Governance
On track	Afghanistan			
	Bangladesh			
	Cambodia			
	Ghana			
	Guatemala			
	Indonesia			
	Malawi			
	Peru			
	Turkey			
	Viet Nam			
Insufficient progress	Côte d'Ivoire			
	DRC			
	Egypt			
	Ethiopia			
	India			
	Iraq			
	Kenya			
	Mali			
	Mozambique			
	Myanmar			
	Nepal			
	Nigeria			
	Pakistan			
	Philippines			
	Uganda			
	United Rep. of Tanzania			
	Zambia			
No progress	Burkina Faso			
	Burundi			
	Cameroon			
	Madagascar			
	Niger			
	South Africa			
	Sudan			
	Yemen			

Source: *Poverty Reduction Strategy Papers; **United Nations Development Assistance Framework
"Assessing countries' commitment to accelerate nutrition action demonstrated in PRSPs, UNDAFs and through nutrition governance." Engesveen et al (2009) SCN NEWS 37

How does the SUN Movement work?

The Movement recognizes that malnutrition has multiple causes. That's why it requires people to work together across sectors to put nutrition into all development efforts.

 Nutrition-specific interventions: Support for exclusive breastfeeding up to 6 months of age and continued breastfeeding together with appropriate and nutritious food up to 2 years of age, fortification of foods, micronutrient supplementation, treatment of severe malnutrition

 Agriculture: Making nutritious food more accessible to everyone, and supporting small farms as a source of income for women and families

 Clean Water and Sanitation: Improving access to reduce infection and disease

 Education and Employment: Making sure children have the energy that they need to learn and earn sufficient income as adults

 Health Care: Improving access to services to ensure that women and children stay healthy

 Support for Resilience: Establishing a stronger, healthier population and sustained prosperity to better endure emergencies and conflicts

 And at the core of all efforts, women are empowered to be leaders in their families and communities, leading the way to a healthier and stronger world.

What worked: Thailand's big push

Thailand outlined their first multi-sectoral nutrition policy in 1977, under the national economic and social development plan (1977–1982). One of the early key messages was that malnutrition should not be perceived as simply a health problem, but should be regarded also as a social and economic problem with human impact. The policy stated that investment in nutrition would not be a short term 'fix', but a national investment for intermediate and long-term growth. In addition, it was agreed that "nutritional literacy should be an integral part of planning and implementing nutrition programs."

Establishing a multi-sectoral policy and plan was the first and major step in nutrition improvement efforts. The challenge was then to implement the program in an integrated manner. The fifth national development plan, Thailand's "Poverty Alleviation Plan (PAP)" was a spearhead of the rural development program, focusing on poverty stricken areas. Nutrition programs were employed as stopgap measures to relieve the most severe forms of malnutrition until systematic solutions could bring about long-term, sustainable improvement.

The PAP was one of Thailand's first efforts to bring about effective and efficient infrastructural reforms conducive to rural development. Effective organizational structure and managerial mechanisms to coordinate and integrate multi-sectoral efforts at various administrative levels and within the communities was critical. Four major ministries, i.e., Health, Agriculture, Education, and Interior (Community Development Unit), were involved and streamlined the integrated budgetary allocations to target poor villages. Each ministry also strengthened the intra-sectoral collaboration among its various departments or divisions.

PAP employed four key programs, namely, (1) *Rural Job Creation* to create jobs for rural people during the dry season so that they remain in the communities and participate in community development; (2) *Village Development Projects* included village fish ponds, water sources and other development projects to improve economic status and household food security; (3) *Provision of Basic Services*, i.e., health facilities and health services; and (4) *Agricultural Production Programs* including nutritious food production (e.g., crops for producing complementary foods), upland rice improvement and a soil improvement project.

Income generation and household food security were the direct benefits.

During the five years of PAP, 32 development projects were implemented in 12,562 poor villages in 38 provinces. By 1986, 550,000 village primary healthcare volunteers were trained, covering almost every rural village in the country. Nutrition activities were integrated within the PHC with other health services. The PHC movement mobilized the community to address malnutrition. It was recognized that successful nutrition programs should not be centrally planned and made into ready-made packages. Rather, they should serve as guidelines.

Another major breakthrough in nutrition governance was the adoption of the Basic Minimum Needs (BMN) approach in village-based social planning, empowering villagers in decision making using BMN indicators in problem identification and prioritization. This was a key contributor to reduction in malnutrition.

In nutrition governance, policies such as primary healthcare and poverty eradication are as relevant as food and nutrition policies. Community-based nutrition intervention programs have a better chance of sustainability if the people themselves become agents of change and if certain elements are in place: community organization for planning and management; community manpower development based on appropriate technology and information and a viable self-perpetuating community financing scheme.

*(**Source:** Abridged from Keynote Talk on 'Thailand's Community-Based Nutrition Improvement' by Pattanee Winichagoon, at the 'Leveraging Agriculture for Improving Nutrition and Health' International Conference, 2011, Delhi, India)*

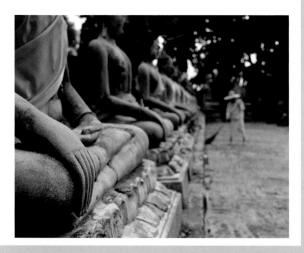

Case study

Scaling up nutrition in Bangladesh

There has been rapid economic growth and substantial poverty reduction in Bangladesh over the past two decades. Poverty rates declined by 8 percent between 2005 and 2010, per capita GDP doubled from 1990 to 2010, and agricultural growth averaged 3.3 percent, due to impressive gains in rice yields (FAO 2012). In line with the Millennium Development Goals (MDG), current estimates suggest that Bangladesh has achieved a 50 percent reduction in undernourishment, will achieve the same for underweight, has achieved the required child mortality figures, and will achieve the target for maternal health. It has also performed well in terms of nutrition improvements, particularly in the 1990s. While progress reduced between 1999 and 2004, it improved again from then onwards.

There are other figures released, highlighting the various success stories. For example, literacy rates for young

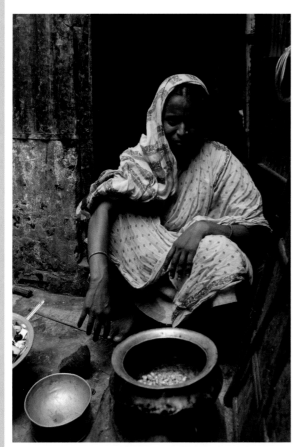

females aged 15–24 years are said to have doubled, rising from 38 percent in 1991 to 77 percent in 2009. Also the coverage of vitamin A supplements for children is now nearly universal, the use of oral hydration salts has increased, and there has been a substantial rise in exclusive breastfeeding during the first six months of life, from 43 percent in 2007 to 64 percent in 2011. There have been several government initiatives that have helped to arrive at these figures, with research and surveys to identify where continued development is needed.

For example, it is acknowledged that nearly one third of women in Bangladesh are undernourished still, and there are challenges regarding population growth, crop vulnerability, poverty and natural resources. Malnutrition in Bangladesh costs an estimated US$1 billion a year in lost economic productivity, there are known to be widespread vitamin A, iron and zinc deficiencies, and cases of anemia remain strong in groups of young children, adolescent girls and pregnant women.

As a member of the Scaling Up Nutrition (SUN) Movement, the Government of Bangladesh (GoB) is recognized for its commitment to improving nutrition. Various initiatives have been launched since 1995, with the current Health, Population and Nutrition Sector Development Program planned to run until 2016, at which point it will be reviewed and updated.

The GoB has mainstreamed nutrition within the existing health system, with improved access to nutrition interventions for those in remote areas. There is a strong focus on the first 1,000 days of a child's life through education and support, with infant and young child feeding schemes throughout the country, as well as substantial investments in agriculture and health.

Specific programs operated by the GoB include the Vulnerable Group Distribution (VGD) and Vulnerable Group Feeding (VGF) schemes, which distribute food items at subsidized rates, based on a rationing system. The VGF program helps those who find it difficult to meet the basic needs for survival, providing food to low-income groups, and VGD promotes self-reliance amongst women. A school feeding initiative has also been started in poor areas with help from the World Food Program, providing high-energy biscuits to children.

Source: *The Hunger And Nutrition Commitment Index (HANCI 2012): Measuring the Political Commitment to Reduce Hunger and Undernutrition in Developing Countries, Dolf te Lintelo, Lawrence Haddad, Rajith Lakshman and Karine Gatellier, Institute of Development Studies, UK, April 2013*

Case study

Global governance: the rising of the SUN

A number of factors served as background to the launching of the Scaling Up Nutrition (SUN) Framework and Roadmap in 2010. These factors include the recognition of the importance of early childhood nutrition, the increased political support for nutrition as being central to development strategy, and the acknowledgement that a wide range of stakeholders, including governments, civil society and the private sector, needed to collaborate if significant advances in improving nutrition were to be achieved.

The SUN Movement is founded on the principle that all people have the right to food and good nutrition. It unites people – from governments, civil society, the UN, donors, businesses and researchers – in a collective effort to improve nutrition.

Following on from the publication of the SUN Framework and Roadmap in 2010, the US and Irish governments committed, in September 2010, to promote the SUN at international level. By the end of 2012, 33 countries had made a commitment to implement the principles and associated programs of the SUN. The Global Movement is supported by a series of Networks, including a Country Network, Civil Society Network, UN System Network, Donor Network and a Business Network. In April 2012, the UN Secretary-General appointed a SUN Lead Group of 27 high-level leaders charged with improving coherence, strategic oversight, resource mobilization and accountability across the Movement.

The key focus of the SUN must be at the national level of the 33 countries committed to the Movement. A particular focus of the Movement is aimed at reducing the level of stunting in these countries. The early indication is that the average annual rate of reduction in stunting in the 33 SUN countries is 1.8%. It is hoped that operational research such as the RAIN project in Zambia – see box – will provide policy insights which can accelerate progress in reducing stunting.

The SUN Movement is defined as "a country-led, global effort to advance health and development through improved nutrition." Not a new institution, organization or fund, SUN is a shared approach that supports the implementation of direct nutrition interventions, while also looking to address the underlying causes of malnutrition and engage the multiple sectors that could contribute to an overall improvement in nutrition, health and development.

SUN represents an unprecedented opportunity for coordination, collaboration, cross-learning and advocacy to catalyze sustainable nutrition gains at national and global levels. Membership of the SUN Movement implies a national commitment to address undernutrition. By July 2013, SUN had grown to include 41 countries committed to scaling up direct nutrition interventions and advancing nutrition-sensitive development, including 18 of the 31 highest burden countries.

In broad terms, the roles and responsibilities of "SUN members" are first, that countries are in the lead and must work to establish coordinated national plans of action, allocate national resources to nutrition and foster a policy environment supportive of nutrition goals. Second, supporters align with this approach by committing to back country-developed plans and build coordination and alignment to leverage resources, knowledge and capacity in a more effective and efficient manner.

The intended "value-added" of the SUN approach is to create a platform to bring governments, businesses and other entities together, both globally and nationally, to find new opportunities to advance nutrition by determining best practices, tracking the effectiveness of efforts, promoting cross-sector learning and strengthening the enabling environment – and ultimately by aligning stakeholders behind a shared goal. A strength of the movement is the depth of expertise and experience represented by the more than 100 organizations and entities that have endorsed the SUN Framework. The collective ability, resources and reach of these supporters has the potential to impact far more communities and nations than any one group could alone. Working toward a common goal through a shared platform such as SUN, stakeholders have an opportunity to maximize the effectiveness of actions and investments.

As it reaches its third birthday, the SUN Movement is well aware that it needs to progressively increase the focus on results on the ground. The success of high-level discourse and commitments made by politicians from the podium can only be judged by their impact on the lives of nutritionally vulnerable young children and women.

For more, please see: *www.scalingupnutrition.org*

The SUN approach

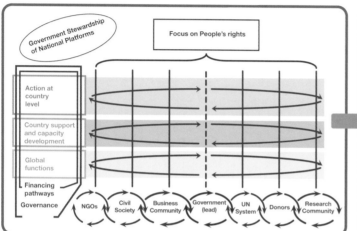

Government Stewardship of National Platforms

Focus on People's rights

Action at country level

Country support and capacity development

Global functions

Financing pathways

Governance

NGOs · Civil Society · Business Community · Government (lead) · UN System · Donors · Research Community

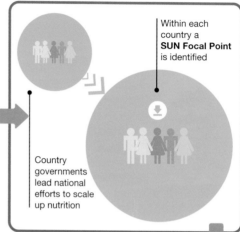

Within each country a **SUN Focal Point** is identified

Country governments lead national efforts to scale up nutrition

The multi-stakeholder platform

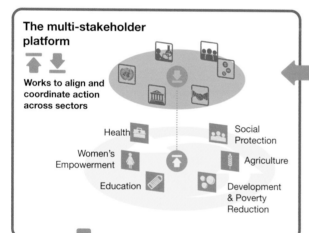

Works to align and coordinate action across sectors

Health

Women's Empowerment

Education

Social Protection

Agriculture

Development & Poverty Reduction

The Focal Point brings people together in a **multi-stakeholder platform**

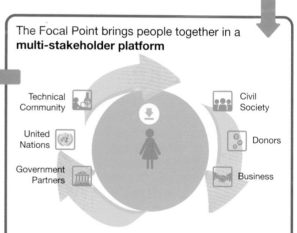

Technical Community

United Nations

Government Partners

Civil Society

Donors

Business

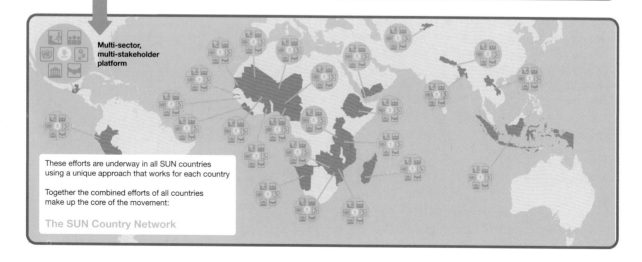

Multi-sector, multi-stakeholder platform

These efforts are underway in all SUN countries using a unique approach that works for each country

Together the combined efforts of all countries make up the core of the movement:

The SUN Country Network

My personal view

Stuart Gillespie

Senior Research Fellow, Poverty, Health and Nutrition
Division, International Food Policy Research Institute (IFPRI)
CEO of the Transform Nutrition Research Program
Consortium. Currently based in Brighton, UK

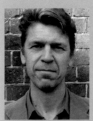 In the last five years momentum has
been building and malnutrition is
finally being taken seriously as a
major development challenge. At long
last there is a degree of harmony with
regard to the scaling up of nutrition-
specific and nutrition-sensitive
actions, driven and supported by
enabling political and policy environments. Various
actors and organizations are converging on the core
challenge and developing partnerships and
collaborations. The energy of the SUN Movement –
which would probably not have survived ten years ago
– is driving this momentum and raising the stakes. As
the political and multisectoral nature of the challenge
is taken on board, issues of governance become ever
more prominent.

Research is more operational and more policy-relevant
than before. In the past, nutritionists did their research,
made recommendations and then implored politicians to
do the right thing. More often than not, it didn't happen.
Now, there is a new focus on opening up the black box
of "political will" to better understand (and ultimately
shape) governance and policy processes, to make
nutrition outcomes, and the policy pathways that lead to
them, more visible.

In reality, political will is a political *choice* – to act to
ensure children grow healthily, or not to act. New tools
and indices and greater access to information for more
stakeholders will help to continue to shine a light on
governance systems at different levels. In this way,
political leaders will increasingly be held to account if
they choose not to act, and they stand to reap the
rewards if they do.

Further reading

Gillespie S, Haddad L, Mannar V. *The politics of
reducing malnutrition: Building commitment and
accelerating impact. Maternal and Child Nutrition.
The Lancet Series, 2013.*

Pelletier DL, Frongillo EA, Gervais S et al. *Nutrition
agenda setting, policy formulation and implementation:
Lessons from the mainstreaming nutrition initiative.
Health Policy Plan 2012;27:19–31.*

Garrett JL, Natalicchio M. *Working multisectorally
in nutrition: Principles, practices, and case studies.
IFPRI research monograph, 2010.*

Gillespie SR, McLachlan M, Shrimpton, R.
*Combating malnutrition: Time to act. Washington
DC: World Bank, 2003.*

Mejia Acosta A, Fanzo J. *Fighting maternal and child
malnutrition: analysing the political and institutional
determinants of delivering a national multisectoral
response in six countries. A synthesis paper. Brighton,
UK: Institute of Development Studies, 2012.*

Chapter Ten

The Power of Advocacy

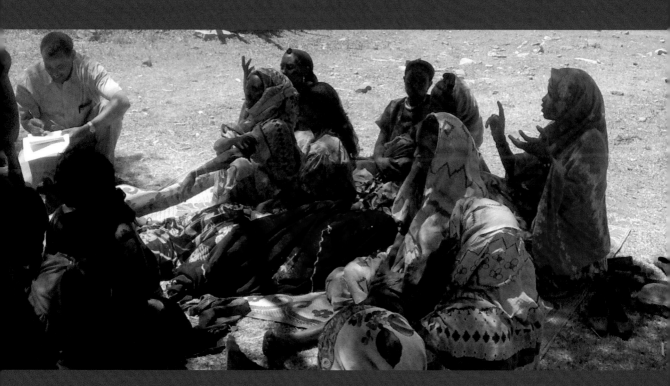

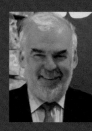

Tom Arnold

Member of Lead Group of SUN
Former CEO Concern Worldwide

"The day hunger is eradicated from the earth, there will be the greatest spiritual explosion the world has ever known. Humanity cannot imagine the joy that will burst into the world on the day of that great revolution." **Federico Garcia Lorca,** *Spanish poet and dramatist (1889–1938)*

Key messages

- Advocacy is a key tool in the battle against malnutrition.

- Advocacy requires a solid evidential base in order to succeed.

- The ability to present a case in powerful and simple language is one of the prerequisites for effective advocacy.

- Advocacy is important, but acting on it is even more so.

- There will be a great work of advocacy to be done in the decades to come.

Food and nutrition security have moved to the political center stage over recent years, both at national and international level. This chapter attempts to identify the key political factors, the changing policy landscape and the people which and who have brought this about. The particular focus of the chapter is the role and power of advocacy in changing politics and policy. But while advocacy has played an important role in this change, it is the combination of shifting political priorities in response to changes in the real world; evidence which demonstrates costs and benefits of particular policies; insights into how policy can be more effective; and the influence and use of power by individuals which bring about real change.

I would like to try to identify some of the most significant factors which have led to food and nutrition security becoming a more important political issue in recent years. This is not the definitive story: that would require a longer and more comprehensive narrative. This is my subjective and selective account of some of the main political and policy milestones which have got us to where we are.

The politics

In 2008 food price riots occurred in over thirty countries. This was the flashpoint which led to food security receiving more serious political attention. The last time food security was high on the political agenda was in the early 1970s when a combination of crop failures, low stock levels and the first Middle East oil crisis drove world food prices to unprecedented levels. But between 1974 and 2005, the FAO index of real – inflation adjusted – food prices fell by 75%.

The simple explanation for this steady fall in real food prices was that supply on world markets outpaced demand and prices fell. The increased supply was due to the increased agricultural productivity from the Green Revolution, mainly in Asia, and subsidized production from the developed world which was exported to world markets. One consequence of steadily falling food prices was that many governments began to take food security for granted, investment in agriculture declined and aid programs for agriculture were reduced.

The last two decades of the 20th century saw big changes in the global food economy, as economic growth rates in China and India increased, bringing significant increases in the demand for food and changes in food consumption patterns. At the same time, agricultural productivity slowed, both in developing and developed countries. These trends led to tighter and more volatile food markets during the

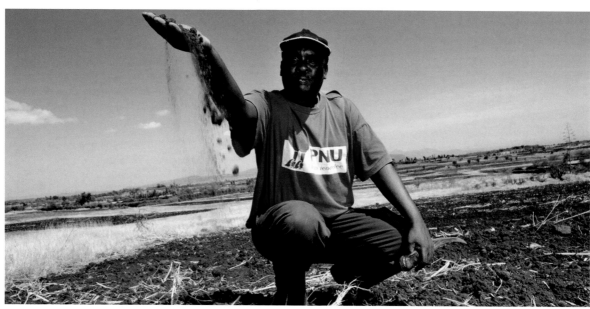

A farmer in Kenya
Source: CIAT

first decade of the 21st century, a situation accentuated by severe weather events in some of the main agricultural exporting countries.

World food prices increased dramatically in the 2005–2008 period, starting with a moderate upward trend until early 2007, and then accelerating to a peak in mid-2008. Prices of cereals more than doubled during this time while the price of rice doubled over a four month period in 2008. The price of key inputs, particularly fertilizer, and fuel prices increased fourfold in 2008.

This was the background which required political action and policy change. In April 2008, the UN Secretary-General, Ban Ki-moon, established a High Level Task Force on Global Food Security, led by Dr David Nabarro, to provide leadership and a coherent UN policy response to the food price crisis. The Task Force produced the Comprehensive Framework for Action (CFA), proposing a set of short- and longer-term policy measures needed to respond to the food price crisis. The World Bank, the EU and the 2008 G8 Summit all took action during 2008 through increased investment in agriculture.

In early 2009, the incoming Obama Administration increased the political prioritization for agriculture and food security. It introduced 'Feed the Future', a program aimed at increasing food security in its partner countries, as a priority USAID program. A further important influencer of policy within the Obama Administration was Secretary of State Hillary Clinton,

who took a significant interest in early childhood nutrition, particularly in promoting better nutrition for pregnant women and for children up to two years, the so-called crucial 1,000 day 'window of opportunity'.

The G8 Summit meeting in L'Aquila, Italy, in 2009 adopted a major package valued at US$20 billion aimed at increasing global food security. US government leadership was seen to be important in reaching agreement on this, but there was also strong support from the EU and other G8 members.

While there was subsequent criticism that these G8 commitments made in 2009 were not fully delivered upon, the G8 meeting of 2012 in Camp David, USA, returned to the issue when they committed to a New Alliance for Food Security and Nutrition, a partnership involving the G8, a number of African governments and the private sector.

In addition, between 2009 and 2012, a number of the main aid donor nations increased their support for food and nutrition security. Within the EU, the more notable examples of this were the UK, the Netherlands, Spain and Ireland. Canada was another important supporter for change. Over this same period, the evolution of the G20 group of nations brought a potentially important new political grouping, with some significant food producing and exporting countries – for example Brazil and South Africa – into the debate on the global food economy.

131

The changing policy landscape

While the above-mentioned events represent some of the high-level political changes, the policy landscape was also changing in tandem. Indeed some of these policy changes were underway well in advance of the 2008 food price crisis.

The policy changes on which I will focus are the following:

- Significant Policy Change in Africa;

- Changes in Nutrition Policy;

Significant policy change in Africa.

The Green Revolution in the 1960s and 1970s had rescued Asia from the specter of major food shortages and had, arguably, laid some of the foundations for the region's economic development. However, for a variety of reasons, the Green Revolution had little positive impact in sub-Saharan Africa. For the last three decades of the 20th century, African agriculture experienced low productivity growth, inadequate investment and significant neglect from policy-makers and political leaders.

The political recognition that this situation needed to change came in 2003 when an African Union Summit meeting in Mozambique adopted the Maputo Declaration which committed African governments to spend 10 percent of national budgets on agricultural and rural development. Subsequently African leaders adopted the Comprehensive African Agricultural Development Program (CAADP). The goal of CAADP is to contribute to the elimination of hunger and poverty through agricultural development. The aim is that the investment of 10 percent of national budgets for agriculture, allied to improved coordination of efforts, at the continental, regional and national levels, should lead to an annual growth rate of 6 percent in African agriculture by 2015.

In 2006, the Alliance for a Green Revolution in Africa (AGRA) was formed, aimed at increasing African agricultural productivity and production. AGRA is financed by a grant from the Bill and Melinda Gates Foundation and the Rockefeller Foundation. The Board of AGRA is chaired by Kofi Annan, the former UN Secretary-General.

The Copenhagen Consensus is an international project that seeks to establish priorities for advancing global welfare using methodologies based on the theory of welfare economics. The project considers possible solutions to a wide range of problems, presented by experts in each field. These are evaluated and ranked by a panel of leading economists.

The project has held conferences in 2004, 2008, 2009 and 2012. The 2012 conference ranked bundled micronutrient interventions the highest priority and the 2008 report identified supplementing vitamins for undernourished children as the world's best investment.

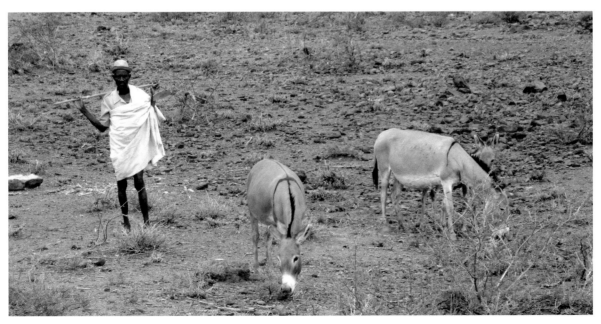

Struggling African farmer
Source: Photo taken in 2010 in Kenya by Klaus Kraemer

The Irish Hunger Task Force

The Irish Hunger Task Force was established by the Irish Government to identify how Ireland's foreign policy and aid budget could have the maximum impact on poverty and hunger. The Task Force started its work in September 2007 and produced its final report in September 2008.

The report examined the particular contribution that Ireland can make in tackling the root causes of hunger, especially in Africa. It concluded that hunger could best be tackled by increasing the productivity of (mainly female) smallholder farmers in Africa; implementing programs focused on maternal and infant undernutrition; and ensuring real political commitment, at national and international levels, to give hunger the absolute priority it deserves.

The report recommended that Ireland, through its government and civil society organizations, should seek to provide leadership on hunger and nutrition issues at international level. The impulse was to try to make Ireland to hunger what Norway was to conflict: Norway has a 50-year history of helping other countries to resolve conflicts peacefully. With a deep folk memory of famine on a national scale, Irish people have a powerful motivation to help other countries combat the scourge of malnutrition; they also have credibility in the eyes of others.

The report was launched at the UN in September 2008 by Taoiseach (Prime Minister) Brian Cowan and UN Secretary-General Ban Ki-moon. In launching it, Taoiseach Cowan said that 'Ireland's history and experience of famine echoes through the generations and influences our approach in helping those with whom we share our humanity in the fight against poverty and hunger'. The report quoted the words uttered by the UN Secretary-General at the High Level Conference on World Food Security held in Rome on June 3, 2008: 'Nothing is more degrading than hunger, especially when man-made. It breeds anger, social disintegration, ill health and economic decline'.

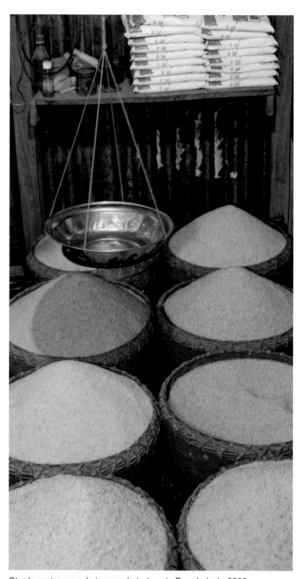

Staple grains on sale in a market place in Bangladesh, 2008
Source: Mike Bloem Photography

The role of advocacy

This chapter has provided a limited narrative about the scale and direction of change in thinking on food and nutrition security over the past decade. Major changes in the global food economy have provided the political backdrop to this. In tandem with these changes, there have been significant shifts in policy, based on evidence that undernutrition had large human and economic costs, and that nutrition interventions provided high economic and social returns.

Advocacy has been a key tool in bringing about these changes. It is much more than simply articulating a case about a specific topic, although the power of reason, analysis and expression is an essential component of it. Advocacy involves articulating a case with a view to achieving a specific change in a proposed direction. More than this, it requires an understanding of the people and organizations that might be able to effect this change, and a grasp of how to communicate with them and engage them for the desired change. Advocacy is therefore more than having a message: it is about understanding how to get that message across and, crucially, following through so that a transformation is indeed achieved. This requires time, a commitment to dialog, and identification of the right people to address.

This chapter has identified a number of the key documents which have been effectively used by advocates in helping to achieve change. The World Bank's policy document in 2006 on repositioning nutrition was very significant, particularly for the focus it gave to the critical importance of good

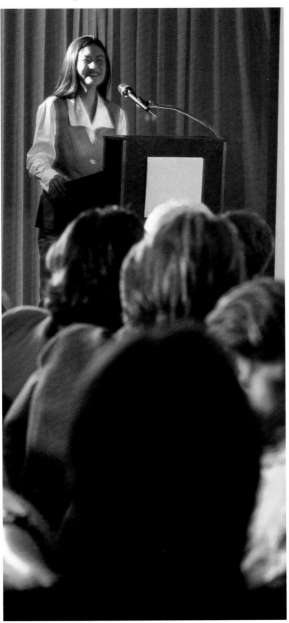

nutrition during pregnancy and the first two years. The Lancet series on nutrition in 2008 gave the world a new way of looking at the subject of dietary intake, particularly among mothers and young children, and a new language in which to discuss it. It also brought home to politicians and policy-makers the scale of the cost of undernutrition and the high economic and social returns of effective nutrition interventions.

The Irish Hunger Task Force report was highly influential for a number of reasons. It was produced at a time, just after the peak of the 2008 food price crisis, when the world was focused on food security. Its recommendations were clear – there should be a greater focus on African smallholder productivity and supporting women farmers: a greater emphasis on nutrition; and that Ireland should play a leadership role in advocacy in the fight against global hunger. The fact that the Irish government accepted that recommendation about its advocacy role was also of considerable importance.

The SUN Movement may indeed be seen as the culmination of many of these separate developments. Although the Movement is not without its critics, it has provided a framework to tackle undernutrition in the countries now committed to it, which involves a range of stakeholders, including governments, donors, civil society and the private sector. In terms of coordination, it has had the benefit of strong leadership from Anthony Lake, the Chair of the Lead Group, and Dr David Nabarro, Coordinator of SUN.

These various developments have also changed the general perception of malnutrition over the past decade. Malnutrition used to be equated in the general imagination with starvation. In fact, starvation only accounts for approximately ten percent of the incidence of malnutrition worldwide. The problem of chronic malnutrition is both bigger and more complicated than many had previously thought – bigger in terms of its scale, and longer-lasting in terms of its impact. The world needs to be aware of this, and advocacy has done much to bring about a change of perception on this score.

It is essential to understand that advocacy, while needing a strong evidence base, requires much more than this to be effective. Messages have to be kept simple, clear and to the point, they have to be repeated and repeated, and the impetus for transformation has to be maintained: policies are not changed overnight. Moreover, even when a policy change has been effected, it will not bear fruit without rigorous monitoring. One has to demonstrate whether a changed policy is having the desired results. If it is, it should

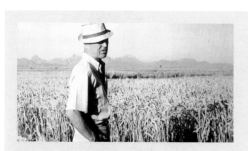

"Civilization as it is known today could not have evolved, nor can it survive, without an adequate food supply."

– *Dr Norman Borlaug*

Norman Borlaug
Source: http://whatsthebigga.blogspot.co.uk/2011/02/greendaddy.html

be further supported. If it is not, it should be adapted or abandoned. Proof of effectiveness is key.

By 2050, we are told the world's population should reach 9 billion, placing greater pressures than ever on water, land and energy. The key international institutions dealing with food and nutrition security – the UN Food and Agriculture Organization, the UN World Food Program, the International Fund for Agricultural Development, the World Bank, the Committee for Food Security – have a profound responsibility to work together to bring about positive change. They are already collaborating more closely than they used to, but this collaboration needs to be greatly intensified, not only with each other but also with donor governments, civil society organizations and leading non-governmental organizations such as Concern Worldwide, Helen Keller International, Bread for the World and Save the Children. There will be a great work of advocacy to be done in the decades to come, using a robust evidence base, simple messages and persistent effort to bring about the necessary changes to the way we live, look after the planet, and feed ourselves.

An exemplary advocate: Norman Borlaug

Widely remembered as the pioneer of the "Green Revolution," Nobel Peace Prize-winning American agricultural scientist Norman Borlaug spent his career seeking ways to improve crop production and fight hunger. The Green Revolution, a series of technological advances that enabled developing nations to improve crop production, often establishing agricultural self-sufficiency, owes much to his revolutionary work.

Of Norwegian descent, Borlaug was born in 1914 on a farm in Iowa, USA. He studied forestry and plant pathology at the University of Minnesota, completing his PhD in plant pathology and genetics there in 1942. After two years as a microbiologist, he signed on to lead the Cooperative Mexican Agricultural Program's wheat improvement efforts with the support of the Mexican government and the Rockefeller Foundation.

It was during his work in Mexico that Borlaug developed new varieties of wheat with special properties. Resistant to disease and high yielding, these were soon introduced in conjunction with cutting-edge agricultural technology not only to Mexico, but also to Pakistan and India, where demand for wheat was reaching alarming highs. In 1967, India imported 18,000 tonnes of improved Mexican wheat seed, with Pakistan following suit. As a result, between 1965 and 1970, the two countries nearly doubled their wheat production, greatly improving food security. Meanwhile, by 1963, Mexico had become a net exporter of wheat.

These remarkable success stories set off what came to be known as the "Green Revolution" – the adoption of improved crop varieties and the integration of new techniques into previous agricultural practice in the developing world. Borlaug himself went on to help apply these methods of increasing food production to other Asian and African nations. The social and economic benefits of this movement were recognized worldwide when the Nobel Peace Prize was awarded to Borlaug in 1970.

Sources:
International Maize and Wheat Improvement Center (CIMMYT), Mexico
http://www.cimmyt.org/en/about-us/who-we-are

Rothamstead Research
http://www.rothamsted.ac.uk/Content.php?Section=AboutUs&Page=Borlaug

The Borlaug Institute
http://borlaug.tamu.edu/about/dr-norman-e-borlaug

135

An inspiration to advocacy: The Great Irish Famine of the 19th century

Ireland's Great Famine, or The Great Hunger, as it is more commonly referred to today, ranks among the worst tragedies in human history. Between 1845 and 1850, approximately 1.5 million Irish citizens died of starvation or malnutrition-related diseases.

The cause of the famine was a deadly new fungus, *Phytophthora infestans* – to which there was then no known antidote – which first attacked and partially destroyed the potato crop in Ireland in late summer 1845. The nation's peasants relied on the potato as their primary food source, and as a result, starved. This blight was to continue over the next several years with the partial failure of the potato crop in 1849, and again in 1850, prolonging the crisis and the suffering into the early 1850s.

By 1855, more than two million people fled Ireland to avoid the fate of those who had died. The population of Ireland, which was close to 8.5 million in 1845, had fallen to 6.6 million by 1851. It would continue to fall – due to relentless emigration – for many decades to come. This decimation of Ireland's population makes Ireland's Great Hunger both the worst chapter in the country's history, and arguably, the single worst catastrophe in 19th century Europe.

Source: http://www.thegreathunger.org/

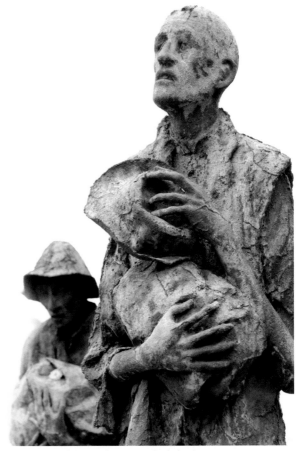

Famine memorial statue in present-day Ireland

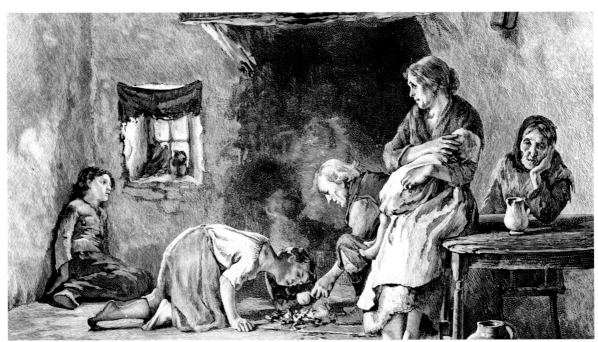

A 19th century depiction of the Irish famine

Case study

An integrated approach to combatting malnutrition

The RAIN Project in Mumbwa District, Zambia

In Zambia, 45% of children below five years of age suffer from chronic malnutrition, or stunting. The Government of Zambia recognizes the importance of prioritizing nutrition, but undernutrition has multi-sectoral causes which traditional impact pathways are often unable to address. The links between nutrition, health, agriculture, food security and livelihoods are well recognized, however, and there is increasing agreement on the importance of multi-sectoral approaches to sustainably address undernutrition.

The RAIN project, based in Zambia's Mumbwa District, Central Province, aims to do just this. By integrating agriculture with nutrition and health interventions at all project levels, it aims to improve nutritional status within the critical 1,000 days from conception until a child reaches its second birthday.

Approximately 3,480 households with pregnant women and/or children below two years of age are eligible. With four intervention wards within Mumbwa District, and two adjacent wards selected as comparison sites, the overall intervention area is randomized into smaller areas that will receive either agriculture and nutrition/health interventions, or agriculture interventions only. Agricultural activities focus on homestead gardening and small-scale animal husbandry; nutrition and health activities focus on behavior change communication for improved child and maternal nutrition, and linkages to the existing health system.

Concern Worldwide Zambia and the International Food Policy Research Institute (IFPRI) collaborated to design and implement this project together with key line ministries, and local NGOs. Irish Aid and the Kerry Group are both project funders. Concern leads the overall implementation, while IFPRI leads the learning and evaluation component and technically supports the integration component. With local support ensuring ownership and sustainability, this is an example of a feasible project model that can be scaled-up and replicated in other areas of Zambia or within the region.

Project title

Realigning Agriculture to Improve Nutrition (RAIN)

Project objective

To develop a sustainable model that integrates and realigns agricultural and nutrition/health interventions to effectively prevent child and maternal undernutrition among rural poor communities, which can be replicated and brought to scale.

Specific objectives

1) To reduce the prevalence of chronic malnutrition among young children and improve the nutritional status of pregnant and lactating women in Mumbwa District through targeted interventions during the first 1,000 days.

2) To realign and integrate activities and mechanisms within the Ministries of Agriculture and Health, especially at District level, to more effectively and efficiently achieve sustainable nutritional outcomes.

3) To use and share evidence generated at the District to influence the local, national and international policy agenda to prevent child stunting.

Target group

Households with children under two years of age, lactating and pregnant women; some activities will include men and the wider community. The RAIN project will ensure the inclusion of extremely poor and vulnerable households.

Number of direct beneficiaries

3,480 households or approximately 20,500 people

Project duration

2011 – 2015

Project area

Nalubanda, Shichanzu, Chona and Milandu Wards in Mumbwa District, Central Province, Zambia

Implementing partners

Ministry of Agriculture and Livestock, Ministry of Health, Mumbwa Child Development Agency, Women for Change, International Food Policy Research Institute (IFPRI), and Concern Worldwide Zambia

Project funding

The overall budget is approximately 3 million euros, which partially is funded by Irish Aid, Kerry Group/Ireland.

Source: RAIN Project Brief no. 1, November 2011

137 **World Population: 1950-2050**

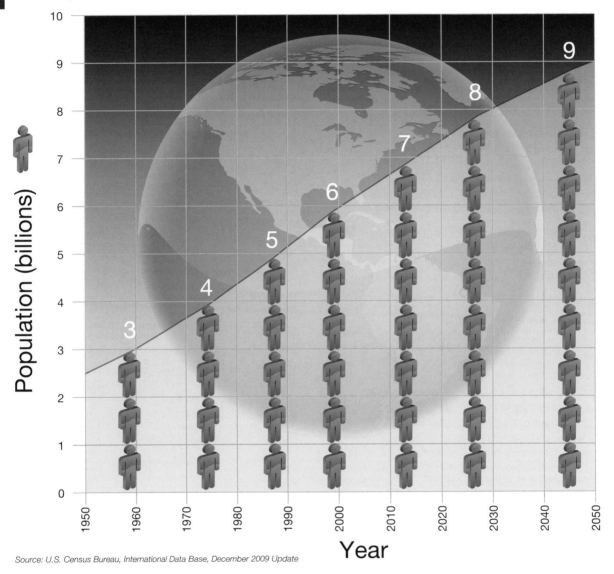

Source: U.S. Census Bureau, International Data Base, December 2009 Update

The growing place of nutrition on the global agenda

1992 – The UN Food and Agricultural Organization's 'World Declaration and Plan of Action for Nutrition'

The World Declaration and Plan of Action for Nutrition arose from the FAO's 1992 International Conference on Nutrition in Rome. Representatives of 159 states declared their determination to eliminate hunger and reduce all forms of malnutrition, stating: "Hunger and malnutrition are unacceptable in a world that has both the knowledge and the resources to end this human catastrophe."

At the conference, delegates came up with a 'Plan of Action for Nutrition' designed to provide guidelines for governments, NGOs, the private sector, local communities and families to help them achieve the outlined objectives. The plan of action contained recommendations on policies, programs and activities resulting from an intensive consultative process.

2000 – The United Nation's Millennium Development Goals

The Millennium Development Goals (MDGs) of the United Nations are eight international development goals to be achieved by the target date of 2015, agreed by all 193 United Nations member states, and the world's leading development institutions.

1. Eradicating extreme poverty and hunger

2. Achieving universal primary education

3. Promoting gender equality and empowering women

4. Reducing child mortality rates

5. Improving maternal health

6. Combating HIV/AIDS, malaria, and other diseases

7. Ensuring environmental sustainability and

8. Developing a global partnership for development

According to the Global Alliance for Improved Nutrition (GAIN), while nutrition is not specifically included within the UN's Millennium Development Goals, it has a direct impact on at least 7 out of the 8.

2008 – The Copenhagen Consensus

The Copenhagen Consensus is a project that exists to establish priorities for advancing global welfare, applying welfare economics to proposed interventions. It has held regular conferences since 2004.

The 2008 Copenhagen Consensus report identified supplementing vitamins for undernourished children as the world's best investment.

The 2012 conference ranked bundled micronutrient interventions as the highest priority and committed US$75 billion over four years to this strategy.

2008 – The Lancet Series on Maternal and Child Undernutrition

The Lancet Series on Maternal and Child Undernutrition in 2008 was a wake-up call for the international community. It stated in its Executive Summary:

"Nutrition is a desperately neglected aspect of maternal, newborn, and child health. The reasons for this neglect are understandable but not justifiable."

The series concluded that a shared approach was needed in order to ensure that nutrition was incorporated into global health and development agendas. It provided an evidence-based call to action, which showed that the first 1,000 days of a child's life are a 'window of opportunity', where actionable nutritional interventions can make a significant difference. Global advocates were able to cite this important evidence to lobby policy-makers and opinion leaders to prioritize and invest in nutrition – this led to the foundation of the Scaling Up Nutrition (SUN) Movement.

2010 – Scaling Up Nutrition (SUN) Movement

The SUN Movement is a response to the evidence-based call to action of the 2008 Lancet Series on Maternal and Child Undernutrition.

In 2010 a diverse coalition including the World Bank, UN agencies and the Centre for Global Development released the 'Scaling Up Nutrition Framework for Action', outlining plans to integrate nutrition interventions and policies across sectors. The SUN Movement now includes 40 countries that could in theory reach an estimated 60 million children.

The SUN Movement is a 'country-led, global effort', focusing on nutrition in the first 1,000 days of a child's life. As its 2012-15 Movement Strategy states:

"Good nutrition in the 1,000 days between pregnancy and a child's second birthday is vital preparation for a healthy adult life with maximum learning and earning potential combined with greatly reduced risk of illnesses like diabetes and heart disease."

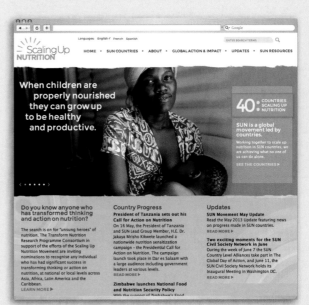

The Scaling Up Nutrition movement brings together governments, non-governmental organizations, academia, business and civil society in a multi-sectoral approach to the problem of malnutrition

139

The 2012 Copenhagen Consensus

The goal of Copenhagen Consensus 2012 was to set priorities among a series of proposals for confronting ten great global challenges. The ten challenge papers, commissioned from acknowledged authorities in each area of policy, included nearly 40 proposals for the panel's consideration. Based on the costs and benefits of the solutions, the panel ranked the proposals in descending order of desirability.

The Copenhagen Consensus 2012 Expert Panel found that fighting malnourishment should be the top priority for policy-makers and philanthropists. Nobel laureate economist Vernon Smith said: "One of the most compelling investments is to get nutrients to the world's undernourished. The benefits from doing so – in terms of increased health, schooling, and productivity – are tremendous."

New research by John Hoddinott et al. of the International Food Policy Research Institute showed that for just $100 per child, interventions including micronutrient provision, complementary foods, treatments for worms and diarrheal diseases, and behavior change programs, could reduce chronic undernutrition by 36 percent in developing countries. Research by Peter Orazem of Iowa State University pointed to the educational benefits of this spending, because malnutrition slows learning.

2012 – The UN Secretary General's High-Level Panel of eminent persons on the post-2015 Development Agenda

In July 2012, Secretary-General Ban Ki-moon announced the 27 members of a High-Level Panel to advise on the global development framework beyond 2015, the target date for the Millennium Development Goals (MDGs). The Panel was co-chaired by President Susilo Bambang Yudhoyono of Indonesia, President Ellen Johnson Sirleaf of Liberia, and Prime Minister David Cameron of the United Kingdom. It includes leaders from civil society, private sector and government.

The Panel was part of the Secretary-General's post-2015 initiative mandated by the 2010 MDG Summit. UN Member States had called for open, inclusive consultations involving civil society, the private sector, academia and research institutions from all regions, in addition to the UN system, to advance the development framework beyond 2015. The work of the Panel reflected new development challenges while also drawing on experience gained in implementing the MDGs, both in terms of results achieved and areas for improvement. The Panel's work was closely coordinated with that of the intergovernmental working group tasked to design sustainable development goals, as agreed at the Rio +20 conference.

Illustrative goals and targets post-2015

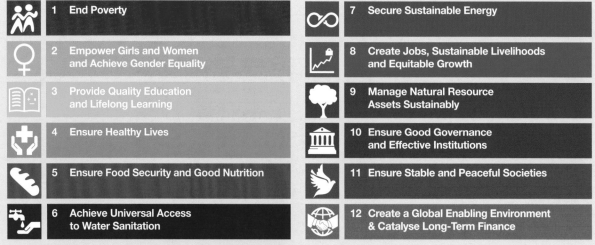

1 End Poverty

2 Empower Girls and Women and Achieve Gender Equality

3 Provide Quality Education and Lifelong Learning

4 Ensure Healthy Lives

5 Ensure Food Security and Good Nutrition

6 Achieve Universal Access to Water Sanitation

7 Secure Sustainable Energy

8 Create Jobs, Sustainable Livelihoods and Equitable Growth

9 Manage Natural Resource Assets Sustainably

10 Ensure Good Governance and Effective Institutions

11 Ensure Stable and Peaceful Societies

12 Create a Global Enabling Environment & Catalyse Long-Term Finance

The report of the High-Level Panel of Eminent persons on the post-2015 Development agenda. http://www.post2015hlp.org/

2013 – The Lancet 2013 Series on Maternal and Child Nutrition

In June 2013, The Lancet published an updated review of the status of maternal and child nutrition worldwide. Five years after the initial series, its authors re-evaluated the problems of maternal and child undernutrition and also examined the growing problems of overweight and obesity for women and children and their consequences in low-income and middle-income countries (LMICs). Many of these countries are said to have the double burden of malnutrition— continued stunting of growth and deficiencies of essential nutrients along with the emerging issue of obesity.

The authors also assessed national progress in nutrition programs and international efforts toward previous recommendations. They observed that: "The nutrition landscape has shifted fundamentally since 2008. The 2008 Series showed that the stewardship of the nutrition system was dysfunctional and deeply fragmented in terms of messaging, priorities, and funding. Much progress has been made since then, largely driven by the new evidence introduced in the 2008 Series, which identified the first 1,000 days of life as the window for outcomes, pinpointed a package of highly effective interventions for reduction of undernutrition, and proposed a group of high-burden countries as priorities for increased investment."

The 2013 Lancet Series on Maternal and Child Undernutrition builds on the ground-breaking work of the series published five years previously
Source: http://www.thelancet.com/series/maternal-and-child-nutrition, June 2013

2013 – Global Nutrition for Growth Compact

In June 2013, UK Prime Minister David Cameron, Brazilian Vice President Michel Temer and the Children's Investment Fund Foundation president Jamie Cooper-Hohn led a high level summit in London of developing and developed nations, businesses, scientific and civil society groups, committing them to supporting a historic reduction in "undernutrition".

The participants – who signed a Global Nutrition for Growth Compact – committed their countries and organizations by 2020 to:

• improving the nutrition of 500 million pregnant women and young children

• reducing the number of children under five who are stunted by an additional 20 million

• saving the lives of at least 1.7 million children by preventing stunting, increasing breastfeeding and better treatment of severe and acute malnutrition

Donors secured new commitments of up to £2.7 billion (US$4.15 billion) to tackle undernutrition up to 2020, £1.5 billion ($2.9 billion) of which is core funding with the remainder secured through matched funding. The UK committed an additional £375 million of core funding and £280 million of matched funding from 2013 to 2020.

Source: https://www.gov.uk/government/news/world-leaders-sign-global-agreement-to-help-beat-hunger-and-malnutrition

141

My personal view

Tom Arnold
Member of Lead Group of SUN
Former CEO Concern Worldwide

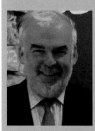 Food and nutrition security has significantly moved up the national and international political agenda in recent years. High food prices in 2007-08 and the political unrest which followed were important factors in this changed prioritization. But strong evidence that inadequate nutrition, particularly for pregnant women and children up to the age of two years, produces physical and mental stunting of children, with long negative long-term human, economic and social costs, has also been influential in changing policy. Drawing on both the changing geopolitics of food and the powerful evidence, effective advocacy has contributed to political and policy change.

This changed environment provides a major opportunity over the coming 5–10 years to make significant inroads in reducing hunger in the world. The latest figures suggest there are 872 million hungry people and 165 million stunted children. An important political and policy mechanism for achieving progress is the Scaling Up Nutrition (SUN) Movement, which brings together governments, civil society, and the private sector to work in a coordinated way to reduce early childhood undernutrition. As at July 2013, 41 countries have committed to scaling up their nutrition efforts, including developing country plans. These plans should reflect political leadership from a high level, as well as engagement with civil society and business, and they should specify the level of financial and human resources necessary. We need to learn what works best across these 41 countries, and to share that learning. Real progress can be made over the next decade if we deliver on what we know is possible.

Further reading

Hunger task force: Report to the Government of Ireland.

Food and Agriculture Organization. The State of Food Insecurity in the World. Rome: FAO 2012.

The SUN Movement website: www.scalingupnutrition.org

UNICEF. Improving Child Nutrition: The achievable imperative for global progress. New York, NY, USA: UNICEF, 2013.

Concern Worldwide website: www.concern.net.

Fan S. 2011 Global Food Policy Report, International Food Policy Research Institute 2012.

Chapter Eleven

The Power of Innovation

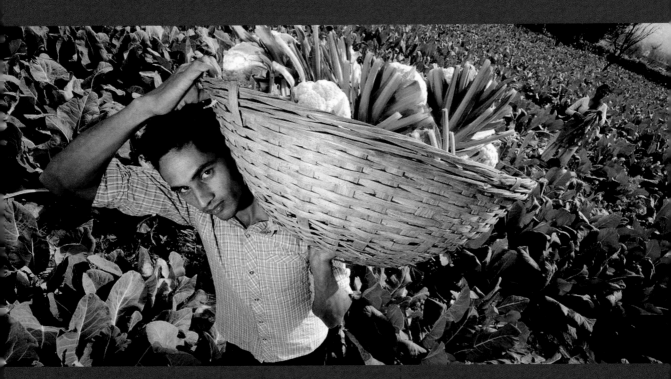

Alain Labrique
Director, JHU Global mHealth Initiative; Assistant Professor, Department of International
Health & Department of Epidemiology
Johns Hopkins Bloomberg School of Public Health
Baltimore, MD, USA

Marguerite B Lucea
Research Associate, Department of Community and Public Health
Johns Hopkins School of Nursing
Baltimore, MD, USA

Alan Dangour
Senior Lecturer, Department of Population Health
London School of Hygiene & Tropical Medicine (LSHTM) London, UK

"Discovery consists of seeing what everybody has seen and thinking what nobody has thought."

Albert von Szent-Gyorgy

Key messages

- For centuries, innovations across the entire span of human nutrition, from plant to population, have targeted aspects of the farm-to-table continuum. Through these innovations, humans have sought ways to improve mechanisms to assess, understand and meet nutritional requirements, both locally and globally.

- Recent transformative innovations targeting distribution systems, leveraging public-private partnerships, and utilizing technological advances have the potential to catalyze research and improve nutrition in both the developed and developing world.

Introduction

In a world of over 7 billion people today, access to sufficient nutrition plays a crucial role in the well-being of the population. Currently, nearly 45 percent of deaths in children under age 5 can be attributed to nutrition-related factors. Others, who are undernourished but survive, face health concerns such as stunted growth and limited neurodevelopment, which impact livelihoods in adulthood. Sir Gordon Conway, one of the world's foremost experts on global food needs, has stated: "Hunger is a daily reality for nearly a billion people. More than six decades after the technological discoveries that led to the Green Revolution aimed at ending world hunger, regular food shortages, malnutrition, and poverty still plague vast parts of the world."

Innovation is essential to alleviate this enormous burden, as it seeks to improve the mechanisms necessary to meet the demands associated with the growth of the world's population and to thwart the morbidity and mortality associated with malnutrition in children and adults.

Innovation in nutrition has occurred since the planting of the first seeds intended to grow food for consumption. In early agricultural societies, the selection of crops directly affected the well-being of local populations, and local solutions were developed for local problems. In the 21st century we live in an interconnected society faced with climate change and an ever-growing population. Increasing yield, enhancing nutritional quality, ensuring diversity of crops and improving access to nutritional interventions have become global priorities. At the same time, we are challenged to define specific nutritional needs and deficiencies at a population level so that programs and policies are responsive to local and regional needs.

This chapter presents examples of innovations that target aspects of the farm-to-table continuum, from plant to population. Recent potentially game-changing innovations are discussed that target distribution systems, leverage public-private partnerships, and utilize technological advances. We first present innovations in production and distribution mechanisms. We then discuss collaborations in the food industry as a mechanism to create an enabling environment for enhanced nutrition. We also review technological innovations that have improved the areas of diagnostics, delivery, and communication. We close with a discussion of new frontiers and directions that further address sustainable nutrition in the world today.

Farm-to-table continuum

The five steps in the farm-to-table continuum provide several access points for nutritional innovations (see Figure 1). Throughout the chapter, we refer to this continuum, in terms of both existing and potential innovations. Many innovations couple one aspect of the continuum with another, illustrating that the innovations along the continuum are most effective when not directed at one aspect in isolation. For ease of reference, each case study title contains the stages along the continuum most relevant to the given innovation.

Production

Farm production is the first stage in the continuum. In the past when facing food deficits, the focus of innovation was on simply producing an increased yield of staple crops such as wheat and rice. However, surpassing the growth of demand with greater production is a necessary but not sufficient response for modern societies. The focus has turned to highlight the nutritional benefits provided with a greater variety and diversity of food as well as the economic enhancement this diversity can bring to individuals, corporations, and governments. In 2011, Rachel Nugent

noted that if farm and food systems are to meet human needs and contribute to human health and longevity, they must produce affordable, diverse, and healthy food. Decision-makers at all levels, both public and private, must participate in steering the food environment in such a direction*. As a consequence, the priority agenda of donors and governments has become one that increases not only the quantity but also the quality and diversity of food production.

As a mechanism for altering food production in a sustainable manner with more nutritional options, some innovations have been developed to combat malnutrition and related health concerns that are specific to certain geographic localities. The first example is the development of β-Carotene-rich orange-flesh sweet potatoes, which have been biofortified through conventional breeding rather than through transgenic approaches. These biofortified potatoes have been introduced in regions with populations suffering from vitamin A deficiency and have been found to be an effective way of reducing deficiencies in women and children (see Case Study 1). A second case study presents an innovation in the fortification of rice (see Case Study 2).

*Souce: *Bringing agriculture to the table, Rachel Nugent, The Chicago Council on Global Affairs, USA, 2011*

The farm to table continuum

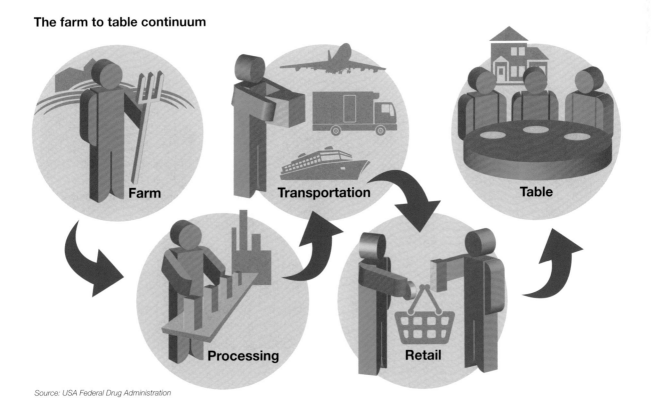

Source: USA Federal Drug Administration

Case study 1

Continuum: Production and Table

β-Carotene rich orange sweet potatoes

Vitamin A deficiency (VAD) is a global problem, estimated to affect over 200 million women and children and to account for over 600,000 deaths globally each year among children under 5 years of age. Deficiency in vitamin A increases the risk of mortality, xerophthalmia and night blindness. Even subclinical deficiency can lead to increased risk for infections, severe diarrhea, and anemia. African regions account for the greatest number of preschoolchildren with night blindness and for more than one quarter of all children with subclinical VAD.

Sweet potato remains a major staple food in several African countries. A preponderance of the varieties grown are white or pale yellow and contain no or relatively little provitamin A carotenoids.In contrast, orange-fleshed varieties of sweet potato (OSP) can contain large amounts of β-Carotene, which is a precursor for vitamin A. Recently several large-scale intervention programs were implemented in Mozambique and Uganda to evaluate the impact of introducing orange sweet potato rich in β-Carotene to rural communities.

Mozambique is a country with modest use of sweet potato as a staple food. A 3-year-long, large-scale intervention in rural communities of Zambezia Province integrated three major components. An agricultural component supported the distribution of vines as planting material for OSP and provided training. A demand creation/behavior change component included education on maternal and child health and nutrition topics targeted to women in participating households and a campaign for the general public to raise awareness of the benefits of OSP as a source of vitamin A through community drama, field-day events and radio spots and programs. A marketing and product development component included training for OSP traders and the establishment of distinct market stalls selling and providing information on OSP. The intervention successfully integrated OSP into the diet of women and children and significantly increased the adequacy of vitamin A intake. No significant differences existed between more or less intensive intervention designs, indicating that future interventions can use less intensive models with the same success.

The large-scale intervention in Uganda resulted in a significant increase in the dietary intake of OSP among children and women in farmer group member households. This resulted in a substantial increase in total vitamin A intake from β-Carotene in all three age groups. It also resulted in a significant decrease in the prevalence of inadequate vitamin A intake among non-breastfed 12-35-month-old children. These children are at elevated risk of VAD, as breast milk is the primary source of vitamin A and the vitamin A requirements for this group are still relatively high; therefore this finding was particularly important. Increased vitamin A intake from OSP led to improved vitamin A status in children and women and reduced the prevalence of marginal vitamin A status in children by nearly 10%.

Because sweet potato is a seasonal crop, this type of intervention will not provide the same amount of additional vitamin A throughout the entire year. However, in these communities, sweet potato is harvested 2 to 3 times per year, and OSP would be available for around 9 to 10 months of the year.

(Sources: 'A large-scale intervention to introduce orange sweet potato in rural Mozambique increases vitamin A intakes among children and women' Christine Hotz, Cornelia Loechl et al. Published in the British Journal of Nutrition, 2011.

'Introduction of β-Carotene-Rich Orange Sweet Potato in Rural Uganda Resulted in Increased Vitamin A Intakes among Children and Women and Improved Vitamin A Status among Children' Christine Hotz, Cornelia Loechle et al. Published in the Journal of Nutrition, 2012.

Low JW, Arimond M, Osman N, Cunguara B, Zano F, Tschirley D. A Food-Based Approach Introducing Orange-Fleshed Sweet Potatoes Increased Vitamin A Intake and Serum Retinol Concentrations in Young Children in Rural Mozambique. Journal of Nutrition. 2007. 137(5):1320-7.)

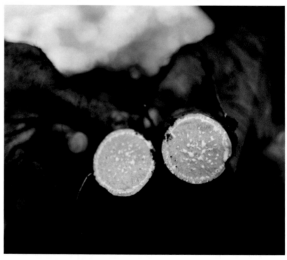

The β-Carotene-rich sweet potato has a characteristic orange-colored flesh

Case study 2

Continuum: Production, Transportation, Retail and Table

Ultra Rice® Technology

PATH is an international nonprofit organization whose work focuses on transforming global health through innovation. The organization's Ultra Rice® technology is designed to be an effective micronutrient delivery system that is culturally appropriate and cost-effective. It uses a warm extrusion process to make rice grains from rice flour fortified with vitamins and minerals, including iron, zinc, thiamin, and folic acid. The extruded grains called Ultra Rice® resemble normal rice in size, shape, and color. When mixed with milled rice, usually at a 1:100 ratio, the fortified rice is nearly identical to traditional rice in smell, taste, and texture. Because the added micronutrients are inside the grains, they are less vulnerable to nutrient loss during preparation and cooking.

In India, a large local miller, Usher Agro, now has the capabilities to produce Ultra Rice®. At the same time, PATH is working within the state systems to widen the distribution of fortified rice within India's public-sector food programs. This work encompasses the Public Distribution System, which provides subsidized commodities to families below the poverty line.

In Brazil, Urbano Agroindustrial is one of the country's largest rice millers. PATH has transferred the Ultra Rice® technology to this miller. In conjunction with the Global Alliance for Improved Nutrition (GAIN), an organization dedicated to fostering private sector investment in adaptation to climate change, PATH and Urbano will be introducing fortified rice through commercial retailers, accompanied by a social marketing campaign to enhance demand for the product.

In Burundi, PATH has partnered with World Vision to distribute fortified rice to children through a school meal program. Supplementing the program, supported by the World Food Program (WFP), with fortified rice aims to improve nutritional status of children who participate. The impact in this country can provide data to support inclusion of Ultra Rice® as an approved commodity for the WFP.

Source: PATH, www.path.org. (June 2012. Ultra Rice® is a registered US trademark of Bon Dente International, Inc.).

NutriRice™ Technology

A similar technology, created by DSM, uses hot extrusion to create fortified rice kernels with encapsulated micronutrients. As compared to some other fortified rice, these grains look, taste and behave exactly like normal rice, and the embedded nutrients are well protected during washing and cooking. The recomposed, vitamin-and mineral-enriched rice kernels have shown demonstrated success in being incorporated into the usual diet. Those ingesting the fortified rice have also seen improvement in health. In Beijing, the Chinese Center for Disease Control and Prevention implemented a pilot project wherein they introduced NutriRice™ into a school's meal plan. The students ate NutriRice™ and vitamin-A-enriched oil and iron-enriched soy sauce for eight months. The students' nutritional condition was improved, and micronutrient deficiencies were reduced by 50%.

Similarly, in Bangalore, India, schoolchildren aged 6-12 participated in a trial of NutriRice™. After six months, the children who were eating NutriRice™ had improved vitamin B levels, and they experienced improvements in physical performance, particularly pertaining to endurance.

Source: A breakthrough in rice fortification http://www.dsm.com/en_US/nip/public/home/pages/productsservices-nutririce.jsp

These case studies illustrate how innovations implemented at the production level can be coupled with enhancements to subsequent steps in the continuum, including processing, transportation, retail and table, to directly address malnutrition. Fortified rice and orange-flesh sweet potato are both good examples of how improved production, in conjunction with robust, targeted population supplementation strategies, stands to increase the pace of progress against malnutrition and its consequences. To bolster the uptake of OSP, production was combined with a marketing strategy for OSP traders, dedicated market stalls for OSP sellers, and community education efforts for consumers. Partnering

UltraRice™ with school meal programs (in Burundi) and government and non-government distribution channels (India and Brazil) coupled production with other components of the continuum. Aiming to establish an agriculture system that is highly productive, stable, resilient and equitable with explicit recognition of the critical role of smallholder agriculture is essential. Small-scale agriculture is once again playing an important role in production that supports diverse food choices and improved nutrition. Women are becoming more prominent players in successful agricultural initiatives. Empowering women in successful farming at local levels improves both their health and their children's health (see Case Study 3).

147 Case study 3

Continuum: Production and Table

Women in small-scale agriculture

Helen Keller International (HKI) is well known in Bangladesh for its homestead food production (HFP) program. The program seeks to improve nutritional outcomes for women and children through promoting small-scale agriculture among women. Nutritional outcomes of interest include dietary diversity and knowledge of maternal self-care and infant/young child feeding practices.

The program was introduced in Bangladesh two decades ago, targeting women with limited land and promoting an integrated package of home gardening, small livestock production, and nutrition education. The program's design specifically seeks to combat micronutrient deficiencies, including vitamin A, brought on by food insecurity and dietary monotony over time.

Project monitoring and evaluation data show that this work has directly benefited more than five million people in rural Bangladesh. Among HFP farmers, vegetable yields have improved greatly. At the "table" stage of the farm-to-table continuum, HFP monitoring has shown a marked increase in the household-level consumption of micronutrient-dense foods, particularly of iron- and vitamin-A-rich dark green leafy vegetables and eggs.

Source: Hillenbrand, Emily (2010). Transforming gender in homestead food production. Gender & Development, 18(3), p411-425.

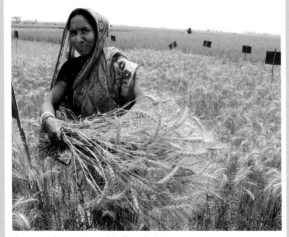

A woman farmer at work in Bangladesh
Source: CIAT

Distribution

Innovations to bridge the gap between production, market availability, and household consumption can improve the diversity of choices available to consumers in remote, rural populations. Yet, distribution is often seen as merely a means to an end rather than a means to grow, develop and innovate in the domain of nutritional access. Yet it is in the phases of the continuum that involve distribution (**processing, transportation, and retail**) where innovation has yielded potentially life-saving initiatives in the field of nutrition.

One of the best illustrations of innovation in the area of distribution also highlights how partnerships can yield untold health and nutritional benefits. In this example, pre-existing private-sector supply chain systems were utilized to deliver health promotion commodities, keeping the costs low but the coverage extensive. The ColaLife project leveraged Coca-Cola's existing distribution systems to piggy-back the distribution of AidPods in a simple, smart manner that ensured oral rehydration kit coverage in the most remote communities in Zambia (see Case Study 4). While oral rehydration could be considered more of a health intervention, similar partnerships could be leveraged to include nutritional products such as micronutrient supplements.

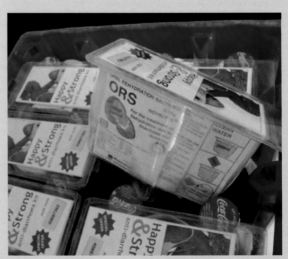

Aidpods utilizing the Coca-Cola distribution system
Source: A Refreshing Development by Andrew Marshall, Development Asia www.development.asia, January–March 2012.

Case study 4

Continuum: Transportation

Medicine via Coca-Cola

"In remote, impoverished places where clean water and medicine are hard to find, people can still buy a Coke. In 1988, when Simon Berry was a British aid worker in Africa, he made two observations that would change his life.

"Fact 1: In remote parts of Zambia, where families scratched out a subsistence living by farming, many young children died of preventable diseases, such as dehydration from diarrhea.

"Fact 2: In these same rural areas, you could almost always buy Coca-Cola."

Berry, then a technical cooperation officer for the British aid program, posed a question of possible connections: "Could Coca-Cola's unrivaled local distribution networks be harnessed to deliver simple but potentially life-saving medicines to hard-to-reach places?"

"Twenty years later, in a concerted attempt to answer that question, Berry and his wife Jane launched an independent non-profit organization called ColaLife. The organization's goal was to leverage Coca-Cola's distribution channels to carry so-called social products – oral rehydration solution (ORS), zinc supplements, water purification tablets – that last mile in an effort to save lives."

They developed the AidPod: a crush resistant, wedge-shaped canister that fits snugly between the necks of the Coca-Cola bottles when in their crates. By using the unused space, the products can reach the same places that Coca-Cola does. Rather than reinventing the process, they found a pre-existing, efficient mechanism to distribute the kits to the most remote of locations.

Source: A Refreshing Development by Andrew Marshall, Development Asia www.development.asia, January–March 2012.

Collaboration

Collaboration between public and private sectors has had an unprecedented global impact on health in areas such as vaccine delivery and medication access, but this synergy has just begun to grow in the field of nutrition. At this point, the potential opportunity for harnessing public-private collaboration exists in several forms, including developing food products and systems, scaling up effective nutrition solutions, providing sustainable cost-effective solutions for information sharing, and conveying much-needed educational messages to consumers. Inroads to improve health and nutrition outcomes could be made on a global scale and can be enacted at all stages of the continuum.

However, these partnerships have been slow to grow. At the Building Effective Partnerships for Improved Nutrition meeting in 2012, companies, donors, researchers, and funders assessed the barriers and explored the potential for innovative partnerships. Several barriers were identified but were not insurmountable, provided buy-in from both sides could be garnered. Partnerships would need to develop shared objectives and mutually meaningful targets. In order to accomplish scalability, the food industry would need to consider corporate social responsibility (CSR) projects as core rather than supplemental strategies. For the partnerships and initiatives to be sustainable, firms need to see a valuable return on investment (ROI) through sustained demand while the public partners would need to see improved health and capacity strengthening at the local level.

Private sector innovations in product development, manufacturing, financial sustainability, message delivery, behavior change and distribution can be applied to public health nutrition strategies. In Case Study 4, a public-private partnership between Coca-Cola and ColaLife has resulted in improved distribution of essential oral rehydration and diarrhea prevention kits. Such a partnership could also be used to distribute interventions more directly relevant to nutrition such as micronutrient supplements.

Successful innovations identify opportunities of value to both the private sector and the public health community. Collaborations between corporations and initiatives for public nutrition expand the value of the corporations' brands and potentially expand the consumer base for the other products manufactured by the company. An important caveat in this realm, however, is the potential for conflict of interest, where public health programs are concerned about exposing already vulnerable populations to commercial exploitation. In an effort to find a more equitable and agreeable bottom-line, an innovative financial model in the private sector is the long-term investment known as 'patient capital', where investors do not expect a quick return on their initial investment (see Case Study 5).

Case study 5

Continuum: Farm

Acumen Fund

Acumen Fund is a venture capital fund that invests in enterprises dedicated to serving poor people in developing countries. Patience regarding the speed in which the ROI is felt has shown to pay off in the long run. Founder and chief executive Jacqueline Novogratz believes that such patience pays, giving the example of an investment Acumen Fund made into an international development project in India.

"In 2002, after nearly ten years of running a nonprofit to help poor farmers in India get the most out of their land, Amitabha Sadangi was frustrated. Government aid to alleviate poverty had largely bypassed individuals earning less than $1 day. Instead, it was subsidizing large farms and being invested in technology he said his farmers didn't want. Sadangi sought to treat the poor as customers, not passive recipients of charity. He decided he would adapt a water-saving drip irrigation system to the specific needs of Indian smallholders and sell it at an affordable price.

"Acumen Fund gave Sadangi's nonprofit International Development Enterprises India a US$100,000 grant and loans to experiment. In 2006, we invested $1 million in equity in Global Easy Water Products (GEWP), a for-profit spinoff Sadangi created in western India to further increase the technology's reach among the poor and sell other products to them.

To date, GEWP and its parent nonprofit have sold irrigation systems to some 350,000 farmers. Including the farmers' family members, roughly 2 million people are now benefiting from higher income levels- for some, $5 to $6 a day instead of $1 to $2. With 101 employees and sales that have tripled since 2008, GEWP is now one of Acumen's most profitable enterprises. It has even begun to pay dividends to its shareholders. By all measures, that is the kind of return on investment we need to see in a world with more than 2 billion people living in poverty."

Source: (Bloomberg Businessweek, The Case for Patient Capital, May 2011, http://www.businessweek.com/smallbiz/content/may2011/sb20110524_877194.htm)

With private-public partnerships, some debate exists over whether patents should be allowed on life-saving food supplements or other innovations. A balance may be able to be achieved if the ROI is sufficient for firms, but not being able to patent an innovation may reduce the incentive to develop such supplements in the private sector.

Technology

In our efforts to satisfy the nutritional needs of the world's growing population, we put significant pressure on the resources of our planet as well as on agricultural systems and distribution networks. At the same time, if nutritional needs of populations are not addressed, the healthcare systems and budgets of nations will come under intense stress as the complications of malnutrition are addressed in acute and chronic care. The systems are interconnected and interdependent. For instance, agricultural systems may be affected by climate extremes (droughts and floods), a deficit of manual labor, a lack of technical resources, or a lack of expertise. Healthcare systems, meanwhile, might be impacted by lack of trained staff and equipment and an influx of patients with nutrition-related illnesses as well as communicable and non-communicable diseases. While technology is not the universal panacea, technological solutions have been developed that have potential to bring about positive and much needed change in several of these systems and at many stages of the farm-to-table continuum.

This section examines technological innovation in terms of diagnostics, treatment and delivery (food fortification, supplementation and increasing dietary diversity), and communications.

Diagnostics

Anticipating complex nutritional emergencies and intervening appropriately depends on accurate and efficient analysis of a population's nutritional status and knowledge of the nutrient content of foods. Understanding potential health consequences of nutritional deficits and how to address them early is crucial in all settings. Preventive treatment can be provided and resources properly allocated when reliable data are available.

Deficiencies of key nutrients such as iron and vitamin A can have dramatic health consequences, severely influencing morbidity and mortality rates of populations. Anemia affects more than 1.6 billion people globally and contributes to at least 100,000 maternal deaths and 157,000 child deaths annually. Vitamin A deficiency affects over 200 million women and children and accounts for over 600,000 deaths globally each year among children under 5 years of age.

At the beginning of the 20th century with the discovery of vitamins, research began on the nutritional composition of foods. Since then, multiple technological innovations in diagnostics have enhanced our ability to analyze the nutrient content of foods, and current methods allow the assessment of several micronutrients rapidly and accurately (see Case Study 6)

Case study 6

Continuum: Farm, Processing, Retail

iCheck and vitamin A

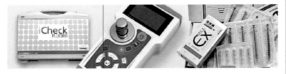

BioAnalyt is a manufacturer of equipment used for analyzing micronutrients in food. It has just created a portable device, the iCheck FLUORO, which determines levels of vitamin A in food. Its use has already been incorporated by non-governmental organizations, the food and food processing industry, laboratories, universities and monitoring agencies. It extracts a sample from any fortified food, such as flour, sugar, or premix, as well as biological fluids, into a disposable extraction vial containing necessary reagents for efficient extraction of vitamin A. Using fluorescence measurement through LED technology accurately determines the vitamin A concentration in food.

The device is said to be as reliable as the gold-standard laboratory-based methods that require significant and costly laboratory equipment and a substantial amount of time. Its portability means that the iCheck FLUORO can be used in multiple sites from the factory production lines to markets in remote areas. The process is user-friendly and the three steps of injection, reaction, and measurement take only a few minutes to complete.

Source: http://www.bioanalyt.com/products/icheck-fluoro-and-iex-nula

Assessing the nutrient content in food is important for the prevention of dietary deficiency, but technological innovations are also required to assess the current nutritional status of populations. Technological advances have been rapid in this area, and include screening diagnostics for both iron and vitamin A status (see Case Study 7a and 7b).

Case study 7a

Continuum: Table

Screening for anemia

A rapid, cost-effective, and culturally acceptable screening mechanism was essential to identify individuals in need of iron supplementation. In recent years, advances in technology have brought about a number of non-invasive screening devices that do not require the traditional blood-draw. For instance, a portable transcutaneous hemoglobin (Hb) meter uses a probe applied to a clean fingertip or arm. The probe emits infra-red light and uses photo-plethysmography and reflectance spectroscopy to establish the Hb absorption pattern in the individual. Crowley and colleagues (2012) tested two similar methods of non-invasive Hb screening and found that both classes of non-invasive Hb recording devices performed acceptably in field conditions.

In keeping with the common phrase, "There's an app for that," a team of biomedical engineering undergraduates at Johns Hopkins University in Baltimore, Maryland, USA, have developed a mobile phone application for screening for anemia. Their 'prick-free' device, the HemoGlobe, converts mobile phones of healthcare workers into 'hemoglobinometers' at a cost of $10-20 per phone. The phone can then read the Hb levels, which are displayed on the cellphone screen. Concurrently, an automated text message sends the data to a central server. The students received seed funding from global health organizations and are currently testing this innovative "app" in the field.

Case study 7b

Continuum: Table

Screening for vitamin A deficiency

Night blindness is a common manifestation of moderate to severe vitamin A deficiency and is also associated with a host of poor health indicators.

In 2008, Congdon and colleagues demonstrated a correlation between serum retinol and pupillary response, advancing work in Dark Adaptometry pioneered by Wald and others in the 1930s. Basically, this earlier work established that individuals with low circulating levels of vitamin A (retinol) frequently suffered from night blindness attributable to associated low levels of rhodopsin, the molecule necessary for vision under low-light conditions. In the 1930s through 1950s a battery of tests were developed to assess, subjectively, the lowest level of light at which dark-adapted individuals could recognize shapes or words. In the 1990s field devices were used in a number of settings to evaluate the threshold of light intensity required for a 'major' pupillary response to be observed; these tests were not practical due to the requirement for dark-room conditions in difficult field settings, but also unpopular due to the subjective nature of the data. In the late 2000s Labrique et al. of the Johns Hopkins Bloomberg School of Public Health developed the Portable Field Dark Adaptometer (PFDA), harnessing digital technology to revitalize these principles.

This new method uses lightweight, head-mounted 'light stimulus and pupillary response' goggles run by a laptop computer to expose participants to a series of calibrated light stimuli and digitally measuring pupillary diameter changes. The device requires no dark room environment and is both novel and time saving, a potential alternative to existing invasive biochemical assessments of vitamin A status which require drawing blood and laboratory analytics. This device is in the process of being validated as a proxy for vitamin A status in a number of South Asian and African populations.

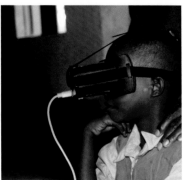

The Portable Field Dark Adaptometer (Labrique, West & Sommer), being validated in Kenyan schoolchildren as a proxy for serum-based assessments of VAD.
2010 Alain B. Labrique

Sources: Validity and correspondence of non-invasively determined hemoglobin concentrations by two trans-cutaneous digital measuring devices. By Caitlin Crowley, Gabriela Montenegro-Buthaneart, Noel W. Solomons and Klaus Schuman.
Article on HemoGlobe innovation, NewsMedical, July 25 2012
An advanced, Portable Field Dark Adaptometer for assessing functional vitamin A deficiency. By Alain B. Labrique, Keith P West Jr, Parul Christian and Alfred Sommer.

While low-cost and accurate screening for key nutrients is a crucial innovation to enhance our ability to respond to the global burden of malnutrition, nutritional status is now widely recognized as the outcome of a highly complex and dynamic body system. The field of nutrition now fully recognizes this complexity and incorporates the fields of proteomics (study of proteins expressed by a person's genes), metabolomics (measurement of metabolites at a cellular level), and nutrigenomics (effects of food on gene expression).

These emerging fields enable us to identify biomarkers, or biological specimens, that can be used as proxy indicators of nutritional status, revealing the intake of food energy, fat, protein, minerals, vitamins, and other components not classed as nutrients. For instance, in the area of anemia prevention, an antimicrobial-like peptide hormone called hepcidin has emerged as the master regulator of iron metabolism, controlling the absorption of dietary iron and the distribution of iron among cell types in the body. Its synthesis is regulated by both iron and innate immunity.

Once low-cost and accurate screening tools for these new biomarkers are developed, major advances in health and nutrition programs may result.

In the field of proteomics, analysis of the entire complement of proteins in cells, tissues, or organisms, has led to the development of diagnostic tests that will not diagnose just one major nutrient deficiency, but have the capacity to assess multiple micronutrient deficiencies in populations. Significant further development is required in this area but such innovations could provide another vital tool with which to tackle nutrient deficiencies.

Everyone should have access to the health benefits of fruit and vegetables
Source: Gates Foundation

Case study 8

Continuum: Table

Proteomics in research and food science

A new proteomics approach utilizing mass-spectrometry technologies is revolutionizing our understanding of diagnostics in food science. The proteome is the complement of proteins expressed at a cellular level and is dynamic and highly positional in character.

Stephen Barnes and Helen Kim pointed out in their 2004 review paper that the study of proteomes and their interaction networks is crucial in understanding biological systems, and tissue and fluid proteomes provide novel biomarkers for the detection and progression of disease. In their conclusion they state:

"Clearly, proteomics and protein mass spectrometry technologies can provide rich resources to investigators in nutrition and related areas of biomedical research. Those who are able to include their technologies in their experiments will make the meaningful contributions over the next decade."

Nutritional scientists recognize the problem of the 'hidden' aspect of micronutrient deficiencies. The new field of proteomics could hold the key. Groups are currently working on establishing the validity of a 'plasma nutriproteome,' which could be the basis for developing tests that assess multiple micronutrient deficiencies in populations on a single methodological platform. Senechal and Kussmann (2011) state the possibilities when they wrote,

"Nutritional proteomics holds great promise to (a) profile and characterize body and dietary proteins, including digestion and absorption of the latter; (b) identify biomarkers of nutritional status and health/ disease conditions; and (c) understand functions of nutrients and other dietary factors in growth, reproduction and health."

Sources: Nutriproteomics: Identifying the Molecular Targets of Nutritive and Non-nutritive Components of the Diet 2004. Stephen Barnes and Helen Kim Assessing Multiple Micronutrient Deficiences In Undernourished Populations Through The Plasma Nutriproteome2010. Ingo Ruczinski, West, Cole et al Nutriproteomics: technologies and applications for identification and quantification of biomarkets and ingredients. 2011. Sandra Senechal and Martin Kussmann

Delivery

Technological advances discussed in this section have more to do with delivery of micronutrients through mechanisms such as biofortification than the enhancement of delivery/ distribution systems discussed previously. Current understanding of the complexity of nutritional processes has led to a significant change in nutritional interventions aiming to improve nutritional status. Improving nutrient intake in this area can occur through nutrient supplementation and food biofortification.

A shift has occurred away from interventions that provide single nutrient supplements and toward those innovations that provide multiple nutrients simultaneously. Industrial food fortification is a convenient method of delivery for multiple nutrient interventions at the population level. Foods such as breakfast cereals, rice, margarine and cooking oils have been targeted for the delivery of multiple micronutrients, with favorable results so far. For instance, Nestle's 'Maggi' cube, fortified with iron and iodine, can be found on the shelves of shops and market stalls throughout West and Central Africa.

Nutrient-dense and safe foods in the form of ready-to-use therapeutic foods (RUTF) are now also being delivered to children suffering from malnutrition. These high-energy nutrientdense foods are typically delivered in small sealed packages and fed directly into the mouths of children. The foods are often made from groundnuts or other locally available staple foods, and mixed with oils and nutrients. One of the first RUTFs to be developed, called Plumpy'nut®, resulted from a public-private partnership (see Case Study 9).

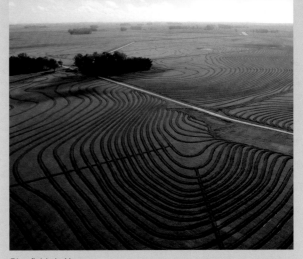

Rice fields in Uruguay
Source: CIAT

Case study 9

Continuum: Retail and Table

Ready-to-use Plumpy'nut®

Plumpy'nut®, a ready-to-use therapeutic food (RUTF), was conceived in 1999. It was developed by a public-private partnership between Nutriset, a French private firm specializing in therapeutic food, and the Institute of Research for Development, a French public research institute. A groundnut-based protein-packed, nutrient-dense paste, Plumpy'nut® needs neither refrigeration nor preparation. The ongoing use of Plumpy'nut® to fight child malnutrition is regarded as a success story in Ethiopia, based on 2008 field research.

A key to its success was the community-based management of its provision, using some existing and some new community networks. Another key was Nutriset's willingness to share knowledge and to allow manufacture through franchises.

However, while Plumpy'nut® was successful in Ethiopia, a 2010 study in a slum area in Dhaka found that eight out of ten women did not like it as a food supplement. This shows the importance of adapting RUTF to the local context for acceptability.

Sources: Management of Moderate Acute Malnutrition with RUTF in Niger. Innovation to Fight Hunger: The case of the Plumpy'nut®. Jose Guimon, University of Madrid. Engy Ali et al, Kamrangirchar Slum

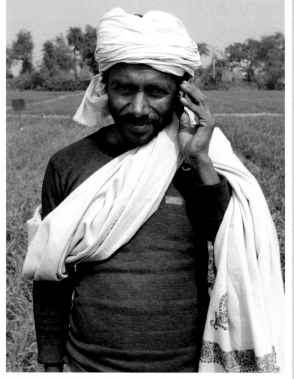

Farmer with his mobile phone in Buhar, India
Source: CIMMYT - TBC

Information & Communications

The global proliferation and widespread reach of mobile phones over the past decade has led to several innovations in information and communication strategies and nutrition. New mobile technologies can be applied in a variety of innovative ways to impact the farm-to-table continuum and beyond, through supporting farming (mAgriculture) and healthcare systems (mHealth).

Applied to mAgriculture, mobile technologies can be used to share important information among farmers. Much like modern agricultural extension which began during the 19th century Irish potato famine when agricultural instructors traveled out to teach farmers about alternate crops, mobile technology has become a 21st century extension worker. It is a mechanism by which essential information can be disseminated in a time-efficient and effective manner.

New technologies have made information more accessible to all, including the smallest scale of farmers. "Plantwise" (www.plantwise.org) is an initiative focused on benefitting small-scale farmers through improving food security for the rural poor by helping them to reduce crop losses. As a modern twist on the 19th and 20th century agriculture extension work, community-based plant clinics share the latest information and research and offer practical advice. The clinics also store feedback information from the farmers in a central knowledge bank. Farmers can access the knowledge bank, which includes information such as the local pest distribution, at the clinic or via a community computer.

Additionally, mobile technology can facilitate the initial steps of getting food from farm-to-table. An illustration in action is the *purjee* system in Bangladesh (see Case Study 10).

Case study 10

Continuum: Farm and Processing

e-Purjee system and sugarcane farmers

Communication is key to successful small-scale agriculture, and in Bangladesh the lives of sugarcane farmers have benefitted from the use of SMS technology. Traditionally, a 'purjee' is a legal permit given to the sugarcane farmers by the sugar mill, informing them that they wish to buy their crops. On receiving it, the farmers then have three days to gather their sugarcane and deliver it to the mill. It is a system that has been in place for over 200 years, since Bangladesh was a British colony.

However, the process has always had flaws. In many cases, the purjees would take more than two days to reach the farmers, who then would not have sufficient time to prepare their crops and bring them to the mills. The purjee system was also fraught with corruption: in the delivery process and in price manipulation.

A system set up as a joint initiative between the Access to Information (A2I) Program at the Bangladesh Prime Minister's Office and the Bangladesh Sugar and Food Industries Corporation (BSFI), known as e-Purjee, intends to resolve some of the issues. Using SMS, the purjee is sent direct to the farmer's mobile phone, along with information on when/where to deliver, how much, and such. The intention with this mobile system is to bypass the myriad problems of the past system.

Source: http://manthanaward.org/section_full_story.asp?id=986

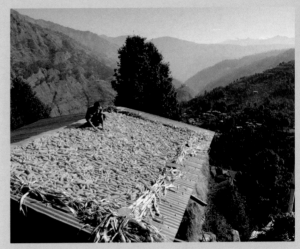
Drying maize in Himachal Pradesh
Source: CIAT

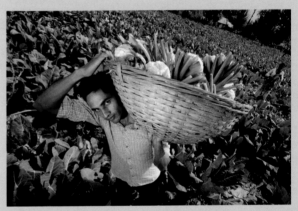
Harvesting cauliflowers in Himachal Pradesh
Source: CIAT

In addition, mobile networks can be mobilized to assist in efficient delivery and distribution of food in crisis situations. Whether helping to organize the multiple actors who are mobilized in times of natural disasters and humanitarian emergencies or simplifying the distribution of emergency foodstuffs, mobile technologies have shown to impact nutrition of those impacted by these situations (see Case Study 11).

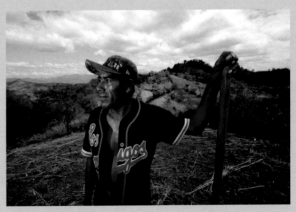
A farmer in Nicaragua
Source: CIAT

155

Case study 11

Continuum: Transportation, "Retail", and Table

Texts and Food Aid

About two million Iraqis have fled their country since 2003, and an additional 60,000 are leaving each month. Prior to the Syrian civil war following the Arab Spring, Syria received the majority of these refugees. At last estimate, there were 1.4 million Iraqis in Syria, many of whom needed food aid, according to the World Food Program (WFP) To meet this need, as part of the WFP program in conjunction with the Syrian Red Crescent, eligible refugee families could receive monthly rations. Each family would receive basic food commodities, such as rice, lentils, and oil, and other items such as sugar, tea, pasta, tomato paste, and bulgur.

As the organization responsible for distribution, WFP alerted eligible families about food rations and directed them to the appropriate distribution centers. Ordinarily, the WFP uses local non-governmental organizations (NGOs) working with the refugees to notify groups when aid became available. However, in this instance, because not all eligible families had regular contact with local NGOs, the strategy needed updating.

In 2007, the UN agency developed and implemented a text messaging program to notify refugees when and where food aid became available. WFP bought text messages in bulk, thereby securing a volume discount, and accessed a list of phone numbers held by the UN High Commissioner for Refugees (UNHCR) to target its text-based food distribution alerts. Initially, text messages to 800 families were piloted. Proving successful in reaching the desired participants, the program expanded dramatically. By the end of the first six months of operation in 2007, 35,000 text messages had reached 140,000 eligible people, the equivalent of one message per WFP-registered family.

Source: Humanitarian Assistance, Wireless Technology for Social Change: Trends in Mobile Use by NGOs.

In the arena of mHealth, mobile systems have also been developed to enhance the capacity of field workers to monitor the growth and nutritional status of children, an outcome of the farm-to-table continuum. The mobile phones have a place in diagnostics and the reporting of screening results (as illustrated in Case Studies 7a and 7b). Information collected can be analyzed immediately to trigger a response, and accumulated data can be aggregated to produce reports for policy decision-makers and program managers.

Another mHealth application is the use of Rapid-SMS, a text-message-based data platform developed by UNICEF and partners, for nutrition surveillance in sub-Saharan Africa. Increasingly used in field settings to support the delivery of interventions, Rapid-SMS allows for monitoring, data collection and information-sharing on a large scale, using mobile telephones. SMS messages have the advantage that they can be sent to multiple recipients, so are ideal for informing a large group very quickly. For data collection, the speed of SMS response means reporting can happen in real time, with no delay while the monitors return from the field. SMS messaging helps information sharing, and the speed means that gaps, for example, in medical supplies or food aid in one area can be identified quickly and also remedied. It is hoped that Rapid-SMS will help to reduce child mortality by shortening the lag time between identifying nutritional emergencies and scaling up treatment in affected areas.

New frontiers

One of the biggest challenges facing the agriculture system currently and looking into the future is how it will respond to climate change. 'Climate-smart agriculture' that increases productivity and resilience to environmental pressures while reducing greenhouse gas emissions requires urgent innovations. The former Director General of the United Nations Food and Agriculture Organization, Jacques Diouf, has given examples of the changes needed to make agriculture climate-smart such as crop diversification, seaweed farming and urban farming, and many of these innovations could be increased in scale in years to come.

The breeding of plant cultivars more able to respond to changing climates may prove a critical innovation for the future. A variety of maize with significantly increased resilience to drought, and a variety of rice able to withstand long periods of flooding (Scuba-rice) are excellent examples of such innovative breeding that are already being used. Some innovations, such as the use of algorithms to provide tailored insurance policies for farmers (see Case Study 12), have yet to be instituted in developing countries, but their potential can already be seen.

consumption present important challenges for the future, requiring continued innovations to develop, produce and deliver optimal nutrition to the continuously expanding human population.

Case study 12

CASE STUDY 12 (Continuum: Farm)

Agriculture and algorithms

In India, where delayed onset of monsoons can bring about crop failure, farmers often struggle to repay the debts they incurred to purchase seeds. More than 15,000 commit suicide every year in desperation. Farming has always been a gamble, but the growing number of unusual weather events, as experts call these changes attributed to global warming, makes seeding, farming, and harvesting an even riskier business.

The Climate Corporation, based in Silicon Valley, wants to reverse the trend and reduce farmers' financial risks by crossing agriculture with information technology's trend of big data. The firm collects all kinds of information, including on weather patterns, climate trends and soil characteristics, and analyses the data down to an individual field. These insights are then used to offer farmers tailored insurance policies against the damage from extreme weather events.

So far, the Climate Corporation offers its policies only in the United States. If its combination of agriculture and algorithms succeeds there, however, it has potential to apply these methods on a global scale. Australia, Canada and Brazil are next on its list of countries to apply the assessments. Perhaps insurance policies based on these kind of analytics will one day also protect Indian farmers against the changing weather patterns.

Source: http://www.economist.com/blogs/schumpeter/2012/11/weather-insurance

Conclusions

Innovations across the entire span of human nutrition, from plant to population, have impacted and improved aspects of the farm-to-table continuum. In doing so, humans have sought ways to improve mechanisms to meet growing nutritional requirements, on local and, more recently, global scales. The game-changing innovations discussed in this chapter target farming and distribution systems, develop collaborations, leverage public-private partnerships and utilize technological advances. They have the potential to improve nutrition in both the developed and developing world. Transformative innovations are often born of interdisciplinary collaboration and increasingly, a 'systems' approach is necessary to address intractable problems in global nutrition. The interdependencies from production to

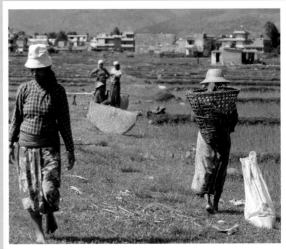
Cattle raised within a silvopastoral system, in which trees are planted at wide spacings into grazed pastures
Source: CIAT

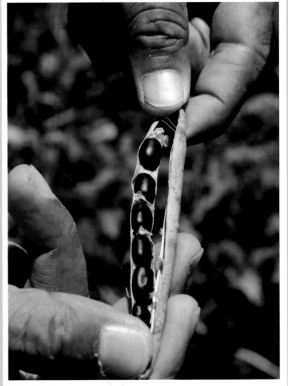
Biofortified beans
Source: CIAT

Our personal view

The process of innovation has been most successful when driven by public health need. Whether in reference to new technologies, transformative methods of cultivation, or simple system processes, innovations that are grounded firmly in the contextual realities of the populations which they aim to serve stand the greatest chance of successful scale. Some have recently criticized the development space as suffering from "technologic solutionism", referring to the tendency of technologies, developed in relatively isolated settings, to search for entrenched problems to solve.

Another often neglected perspective is that of the end-users or beneficiaries of the innovations we seek to develop. Increasingly, researchers are identifying the value of substantial inclusion of these stakeholders in the process of priority-setting, identifying barriers and constraints to optimal outcomes and in the design and implementation of innovations themselves. Not only is the likelihood of achieving better "fit" with the target populations increased, but a local ownership of the strategy is fostered through such methods.

Finally, the importance of continued prioritization and investment in high-quality research cannot be understated. Donors and implementing agencies must focus considerable energy not only on "implementation science", that is exploring how best to deliver what we know is efficacious, but also on developing and testing the efficacy of new solutions. To quote Dean Emeritus Alfred Sommer of the Johns Hopkins Bloomberg School of Public Health, "Today's research forms the basis for tomorrow's programs." Investment is necessary into research that is rigorous, problem-driven, collaborative, interdisciplinary and which seeks to build and engage local capacity.

Further reading

Hilary Green J, Van Bladeren PJ, Bruce German J. *Translating Nutrition Innovation into Practice.* Institute of Food Technologies. *www.ift.org.*

Eggersdorfer M. *Tackling poverty with nutrition innovations.* The Chicago Council on Global Affairs.

Inclusive Agriculture Sector Growth. Feed the Future, the US government's global hunger and food security initiative.

Ash C, Jasny BR, Malakoff DA, Sugden AM. *Feeding the future.* Science Magazine.

Mobile agriculture. Float Mobile Learning website: *floatlearning.com/magriculture*

Brugger F. *Mobile Applications in Agriculture.* Syngenta Foundation.

Woodill G, Udell C. *The Application of Mobile Computing to the Business of Farming.* Float Mobile Learning.

Chapter Twelve

Speaking Up for Nutrition:
The Role of Civil Society

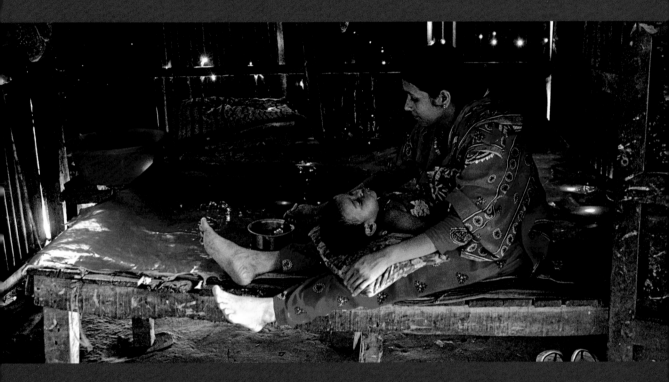

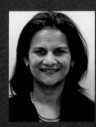

Asma Lateef
Director, Bread for the World Institute
Washington DC, USA

"The evidence is clear that governments can't do this alone. Momentum for improving nutrition is strong, in large part thanks to our civil society partners who have worked tirelessly to mobilize support around the world behind the evidence that nutrition matters."

Rajiv Shah, Administrator, USAID

Key messages

- Civil society has helped to shape the Scaling Up Nutrition (SUN) Movement at global level and helps to deliver improved nutrition at country level.

- As the deadline for the Millennium Development Goals approaches, hunger and malnutrition remain part of the unfinished agenda.

- As the international community debates the post-2015 development framework, food security and nutrition should be explicitly addressed in the goals, and stunting should be a priority indicator.

- Civil society organizations work closely in, and with, communities, and have experience in implementing multi-sectoral programs. They are uniquely positioned to advocate for greater attention to hunger and malnutrition.

- By engaging national governments on the post-2015 agenda, civil society can play an important role in elevating nutrition as a priority for the next set of goals.

From its first beginnings, the Scaling Up Nutrition (SUN) Movement has been a multi-stakeholder effort. Civil society organizations have been engaged in establishing SUN and civil society is represented on the SUN Lead Group.

At the global level, as noted in Chapter 10 of the present volume, civil society has helped shape and build support for SUN with donor governments. At the country level, civil society organizations have an important role to play in strengthening the political will, engaging in policy development/reform; in designing and implementing programs; and in monitoring and feedback.

In June 2011, the first international meeting to help organize the voice of civil society in the SUN Movement was held in Washington. The focus was on building political commitment to scaling up nutrition as part of the 1,000 Days Partnership and Call to Action. Participants discussed the unique role of civil society. Specifically, it was noted that civil society organizations work closely in and with communities. They have extensive reach, often working in areas that are not being served by government programs. They also have a great deal of experience with implementation and a greater understanding of the causes of undernutrition in each community that can and should be leveraged. Participants also noted that civil society organizations work across sectors and have developed integrated solutions in their programs.

Civil society also has an important role to play in advocacy. Political leadership and support is essential to making progress on any given issue. Civil society organizations can help develop leaders and champions and improve the enabling policy environment for addressing maternal and child nutrition through advocacy. They can :

Educate and rally support

- Draw attention to and define the issues;

- Build consensus among other civil society actors and policy advocates;

- Work together to shape and advance policy solutions and recommendations.

Persuade

- Elevate the importance of an issue;

- Urge leadership on an issue;

- Identify and engage effective and credible messengers.

Leverage

- Engage the debates that are happening within or between governmental ministries or departments or between the parliament and the administration;

- Lend support to a specific point of view within the debate and make the case for a specific set of policy solutions.

Broker

- Carry information and messages between different players;

- Help identify common objectives;

- Add pressure when needed or helpful.

Engage and mobilize grassroots constituents

- Inform and educate grassroots and the engaged public about issues – show connections between issues and how specific policy actions can help;

- Demonstrate public support for specific measures being debated;

- Build relationships with members of parliament and their staff – to show that there is a long-term constituency around the issues.

In the two years since the first civil society gathering, there has been much progress in deepening the engagement of civil society in the SUN Movement. To date, 11 SUN country civil society alliances have received funding from donors to support their efforts, including through the SUN's Multi-Partner Trust Fund. In June 2013, the SUN Civil Society Network was launched and held its inaugural meeting alongside a civil-society-led event, Sustaining Political Commitments to Scaling Up Nutrition, to mark the first 1,000 days of SUN and to look ahead to the next 1,000 days. The two events served to highlight some of civil society's successes in elevating nutrition as a priority and in building nutrition champions.

In Peru, a coalition of civil society organizations called the Child Nutrition Initiative (CNI) has worked together to obtain commitments to reduce malnutrition among children under 5 by 5 percent in 5 years from the 10 presidential candidates running in the national elections in 2005 . They followed up with specific recommendations and a 100- day action plan for the newly-elected President Alan Garcia, who pledged to reduce malnutrition by 9 percent. To sustain political commitments, CNI also worked with other stakeholders, regional leaders and the World Bank, to build long-term support and commitment to nutrition. When

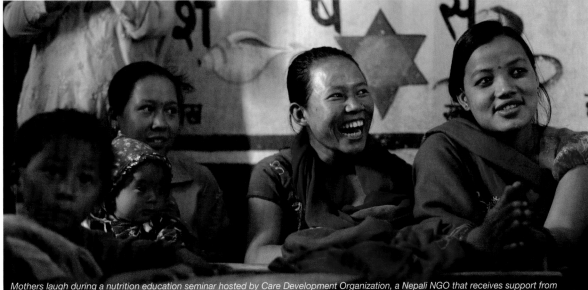

Mothers laugh during a nutrition education seminar hosted by Care Development Organization, a Nepali NGO that receives support from Maryknollers, in Bandarkharka, Nepal, on Friday, April 27, 2012. About 30 women plus their kids and grandkids attended the seminar.

The seminar focused on recognizing the signs of malnutrition in children and learning how to prepare foods hygienically. A health worker taught the women about vaccinations for children, prolapsed uterus and the importance of cutting an umbilical cord with a sterilized knife. She also stressed that children need to be fed multiple times a day, which doesn't always happen since the women labor in fields all day. All produce used in the seminar is locally available.

Photo by Laura Elizabeth Pohl/Bread for the World

161

President Ollanta Humala came into office in 2011, he pledged to continue the commitment to nutrition. He established the Ministry of Development and Social Inclusion (MIDIS), with a specific mandate to coordinate government agencies, private sector and civil society to reduce child chronic malnutrition by 10 percent. The first lady of Peru is on the SUN Lead Group.

Since 2011, civil society organizations in Zambia have helped elevate the issue of maternal and child nutrition as a national priority. In 2012, they have established the Zambia Civil Society Scaling Up Nutrition Alliance (CSO-SUN), which has raised awareness of the impact of chronic maternal and child malnutrition on Zambia's development through the media. The Post Newspaper in Zambia wrote in December 2012 :

"We are told that 45 percent of our children under the age of five – a terrifying percentage – are affected by malnutrition. The painful truth is that, despite the goals to eradicate it, malnutrition among our under-fives still persists and tends to grow. For 45 percent of our children under the age of five, malnutrition is not a mere conceptual reference, but rather a tragic daily experience, a disgraceful reality for

all of us ...This is an affront to our collective conscience. It is an imperative need of our times to be aware of this reality, because of what a situation affecting 45 percent of our children under the age of five entails in terms of human suffering and the squandering of life and intelligence ...We appreciate and exalt the work being done by Zambia Civil Society Scaling up Nutrition Alliance in creating an awareness of the inevitable need for profound socio-economic structural changes that are needed to address these problems."

The editorial went on to call on the government to take action. In February 2013 the civil society alliance hosted a media capacity building workshop to educate journalists on the issue.

In April 2013 the government launched the National Food and Nutrition Strategic Plan 2011– 2015 and the First 1,000 Most Critical Days Program (MCDP). Dr Joseph Katema, Minister of Community Development, Mother and Child Health; Mr Malcom Geere, DfID Deputy Head of Office and representative of the SUN donor convenor in Zambia; and William Chilufya, Coordinator of the CSO-SUN in Zambia spoke at the launch. The alliance's

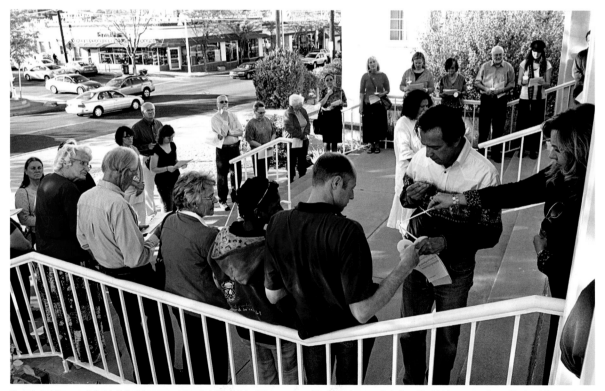

People hold a candlelight vigil at Immanuel Baptist Church in Albuquerque, New Mexico, on October 22, 2011, to pray for a Circle of Protection around US federal programs that help poor and hungry people in the United States and abroad.
Photo by Laura Elizabeth Pohl/Bread for the World

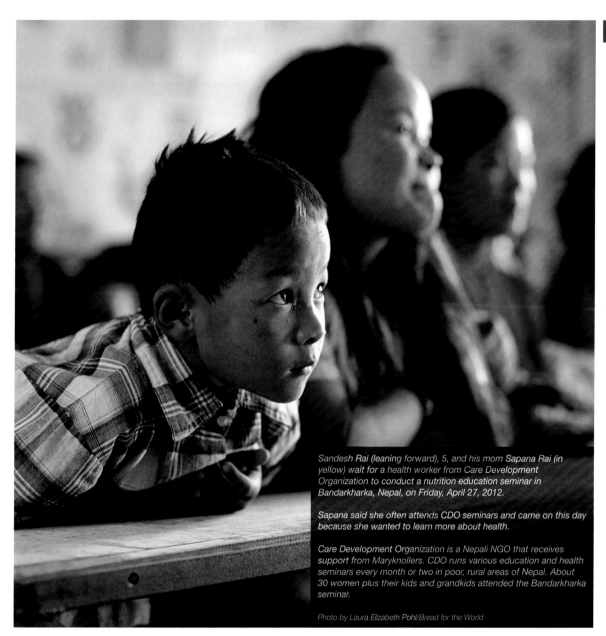

Sandesh Rai (leaning forward), 5, and his mom Sapana Rai (in yellow) wait for a health worker from Care Development Organization to conduct a nutrition education seminar in Bandarkharka, Nepal, on Friday, April 27, 2012.

Sapana said she often attends CDO seminars and came on this day because she wanted to learn more about health.

Care Development Organization is a Nepali NGO that receives support from Maryknollers. CDO runs various education and health seminars every month or two in poor, rural areas of Nepal. About 30 women plus their kids and grandkids attended the Bandarkharka seminar.

Photo by Laura Elizabeth Pohl/Bread for the World

effective advocacy has also succeeded in building champions in the parliament. At the June 2013, Sustaining Political Commitments event, representatives of Zambia's government, parliament and civil society alliance spoke about Zambia's experience in scaling up nutrition.

In Tanzania, the Partnership for Nutrition in Tanzania (PANITA) was launched in 2011. It now includes 280 civil society organization members implementing nutrition programs across Tanzania. PANITA's mission is "to advance advocacy efforts and improve mobilization and coordination of civil society organizations to contribute towards a more effective national and local response to addressing undernutrition.[1] PANITA has engaged 34 members of the Tanzania Union Parliament and House of Representatives in Zanzibar "to act as 'nutrition champions'." It also works with the Tanzania Association of Journalists for Children that represent the 15 major media agencies." PANITA is also represented on Tanzania's High Level Steering Committee on Nutrition.

Nutrition and the Post-2015 Development Agenda – the role of civil society

There is gathering momentum around the post-2015 development agenda. Civil society engaged in nutrition and nutrition advocacy globally and in SUN countries specifically should pay attention to the debate and engage constructively to ensure that nutrition is strongly represented in whatever framework is agreed.

Since 2000, the Millennium Development Goals (MDGs) have been the dominant global development framework. The MDGs have come to represent the most holistic approach yet to human development. They have galvanized public support around the world for ending hunger and extreme poverty. In 2012, the World Bank announced that the percentage of people living below the international poverty line had already fallen by more than half, thus achieving a 2015 target for MDG 1, which calls for cutting extreme poverty and hunger in half. More people escaped poverty during the 2000s than in any decade in history. Even more importantly, progress was made in every major region of the world. In addition, since 1990, the baseline year for measuring progress towards the MDGs, at least 75 percent of all participating countries have made progress in reducing poverty, hunger, and maternal/child mortality, and in providing clean drinking water. Nearly two-thirds of countries have made progress in gender equality by improving girls' enrollment in primary school. Between 1999 and 2005, the number of children dying of measles fell by 75 percent – from more than 500,000 deaths each year to about 126,000. Overall, there has been a two-thirds reduction in child mortality, due largely to the continued rollout of vaccines. Clear, time-bound and measurable targets have certainly been important in focusing political attention and resources on the MDGs and improving accountability for results.

Despite these successes, much remains to be done, and challenges remain. Significantly, hunger and malnutrition are still part of the unfinished agenda. At the current rate of progress, the hunger target will not be met by 2015. The MDGs measure progress in reducing hunger by calorie intake and children's weight. Yet even combining efforts to improve calorie intake and children's weight with the dramatic reduction in extreme poverty that has been achieved has not been effective in speeding up progress against malnutrition, particularly the continued high rates of stunting (when a child is far too short for age) and wasting (when a child weighs far too little for height) - both of which are signs of chronic malnutrition.

Over the next two years, as we approach the MDG deadline of December 2015, it is imperative to invest more resources in strategies to reduce malnutrition that we know to be effective. In 2015, through a process shepherded by the United Nations, national leaders are expected to decide on a new set of global development goals. A vigorous debate about what these goals should be is already under way. There are many ideas now being put forward about what a new set of goals should include. It is critical to include hunger and malnutrition targets. National leaders will identify these based on the recommendations of the international development community, reflecting the best medical and scientific evidence, and there is growing consensus on how to do this.

WHO nutrition targets for 2025

In 2012, the UN World Health Organization (WHO) agreed a set of six nutrition targets to be achieved by 2025. These are:

- A 40 percent reduction in the global number of children under age 5 who are stunted;

- 50 percent reduction in anemia among women of reproductive age;

- 30 percent reduction in low birth weight;

- No increase in childhood overweight;

- An increase to 50 percent in the proportion of infants breastfed exclusively (no other food or water) for the first 6 months.

- A reduction of childhood wasting to 5 percent and maintenance of the rate at 5 percent or lower.

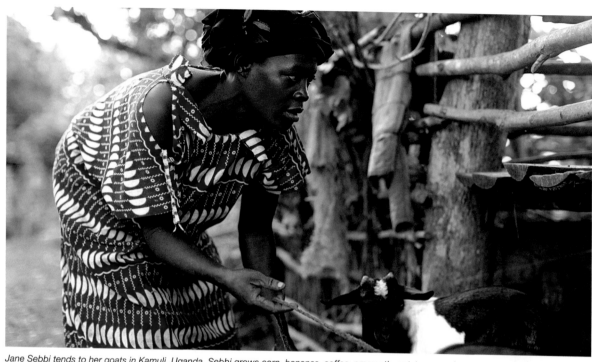

Jane Sebbi tends to her goats in Kamuli, Uganda. Sebbi grows corn, bananas, coffee, amaranth, potatoes, soy beans, common beans and sweet potatoes. She also takes care of pigs, goats and chickens
Photo by Laura Elizabeth Pohl/Bread for the World

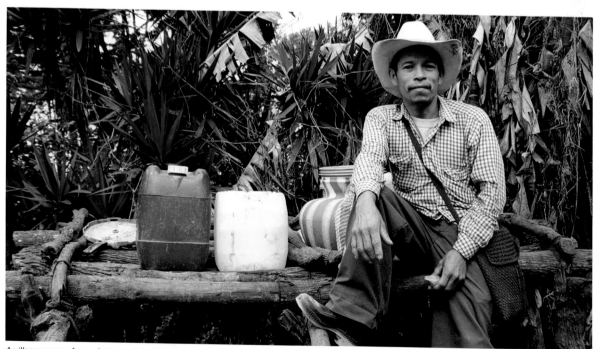

A villager poses for a photograph in Chiquimula, Guatemala. Chiquimila is in the Corredor Seco (Dry Corridor), an area near the Honduran border that recently suffered a severe drought, thus exacerbating poverty and malnutrition in a country that has the highest malnutrition rate in the Western Hemisphere.
Photo by Todd Post/Bread for the World Institute

At a February 2013 consultation on "nutrition in the post-2015 development agenda" in Washington, DC, nutrition experts agreed that nutrition should be more explicitly addressed in the next set of development goals and that stunting should be the priority indicator. Stunting is a powerful indicator, not only of the impact of malnutrition on a child, but also of chronic inequality and deprivation in a community. Experts also agreed that the next set of goals need more than one nutrition indicator, and that the WHO targets provide a sound set of alternatives.

In May 2013, the Report of the High-Level Panel of Eminent Persons on the Post-2015 Development Agenda released their recommendations and illustrative goals and targets . The panel proposed five transformative shifts needed to achieve a more equitable and peaceful world:

leave no one behind, put sustainable development at the core, transform economies for jobs and inclusive growth, build peace and effective open and accountable institutions for all, and forge a new global partnership. In order to achieve these shifts, the panel recommended a set of illustrative goals and targets, including one that would "Ensure Food Security and Good Nutrition."

In September 2013, UN Secretary-General Ban Ki-moon will present his report on the post-2015 agenda. Then, over the next two years, governments will begin to negotiate amongst themselves with the objective of reaching an agreement by 2015. It is crucial at this stage that civil society in all countries engages governments about the importance of a new set of goals and about ensuring that nutrition is integrated into the post-2015 development framework.

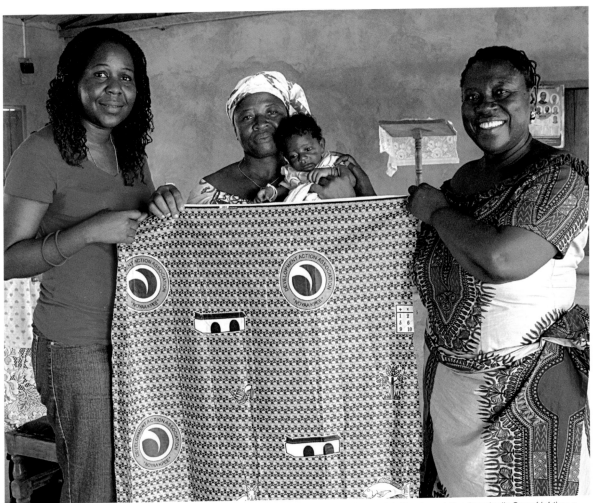

Faustine Wabwire (left) from Bread for the World Institute receives a banner of the Development Action Association from Lydia Sasu (right) as a token appreciation for coming to Ghana and talking with women farmers that DAA has trained.
Photo by Todd Post/Bread for the World Institute

Case study

Guatemala: Gilma's Story

In a country like Guatemala, where social norms change slowly, gender parity in education can't come soon enough. Guatemala is a middle-income country, but it has the highest rate of malnutrition in the Western Hemisphere and one of the highest in the world. It also ranks near the top of an index measuring inequality in Latin America.

Gilma, a five-year-old girl, lives in a Guatemalan village precariously on the edge of food insecurity in the best of times. In more challenging times, children like her are at grave risk. In 2011, a severe drought struck her region of the country, leading the US government to send food aid. Without the food aid, many children there might have died from malnutrition, and this is what almost happened to Gilma.

Gilma has four siblings, all of them boys, and that means she and her mother eat last and often there is nothing left for them. Her greatest disadvantage is not that she is a poor child in a region where food is often scarce, but that she is a poor girl there. By November 2011, Gilma was suffering from a condition known as severe acute malnutrition (SAM). Her legs were swollen and ulcerated, as happens when children suffer such severe malnutrition. In Guatemala, when a child falls below the SAM threshold, government health officials must be alerted and they will then assume responsibility for care.

Gilma was fortunate in that her village was receiving food aid. Save the Children, the nongovernmental organization (NGO) administering the program, contacted health officials when Gilma slipped from moderate to severe acute malnutrition, but the officials didn't respond right away. She is alive today because of the persistence of Save the Children staff in getting the officials' attention.

Before long, Gilma will be going to school; hopefully, her education will enable her to prevent what happened to her from happening to her daughters.

Source: Bread for the World 2013 Hunger Report

Case study

Ghana: Lydia's Story

The Development Action Association (DAA) provides training to women farmers in Ghana, working in some of the poorest communities in the country. Lydia Sasu is the executive director of DAA, which she co-founded in 1997. Before DAA, Ms Sasu worked in Ghana's Ministry of Agriculture and served as the country's first female agriculture extension agent. Working with women farmers has been her life's work, shaped by her experiences as a child watching her mother struggle against obstacles that have hardly changed for the women she works with today.

In spite of the success Ghana has had in reducing hunger - meeting the 2015 MDG target before any other country in sub-Saharan Africa - progress has not been shared equally by all. Rural women and girls are the most disadvantaged members of society. This remains true of Ghana, even though its record of progress on gender equality is stronger than that of many other African countries. Progress on the MDGs is bound to stall until it is a top priority to confront and correct the structural inequalities that hold marginalized groups in society back.

In recent years, Sasu, now 65, has been invited to speak at international events on women in agriculture, most recently at the United Nations on International Women's Day 2012. UN Secretary-General Ban Ki-moon has pledged to incorporate consultations with multiple stakeholders into efforts to develop post-2015 global development goals. Consultations are planned in 50 countries and are supposed to include civil society organizations such as DAA. The participation of civil society is critical in developing a post-2015 development consensus that reflects the views of poor and hungry people themselves.

Source: Bread for the World 2013 Hunger Report

167

Case study

Bangladesh: Tohomina's Story

The afternoon hours are Tohomina Akter's favorite time of day. That's when she can take a break from her household tasks, rest, and play with her 17-month-old daughter, Adia. Like any toddler, Adia much prefers movement.

Adia runs through the four rooms of their home, her pink sundress and plastic pink shoes contrasting against the gray tin walls. First is her parent's bedroom, then the room where her father's parents and brothers sleep. Then a small room that contains clothes and dishes, and finally the kitchen, a skinny corridor that opens to the outside on one end, where her mother prepares their food over a fire.

Adia stops suddenly at the front steps, looking out at the familiar faces of Char Baria, a village in the Barisal district of Bangladesh. In front of her lies Tohomina's garden, a 25-foot square of spinach, amaranth, chili, and pepper plants, an important source of nutrients for Adia and her family. Spinach and red amaranth are Adia's favorites.

Tohomina planted the garden after receiving training in "Nobo Jibon," a program administered by Helen Keller International, a nongovernmental organization that works in several Bangladesh districts. The vegetables she harvests have increased the nutrients available to her family, especially her daughter. What's more, the extra money the family earns selling the surplus vegetables goes toward buying additional food for Adia.

In the program, Tohomina learned why a diverse, healthy diet is important, and also about the importance of breastfeeding her daughter. Tohomina attended classes for almost two months, hearing from health workers the benefits of giving Adia only breast milk during her first six months of life.

Tohomina has stuck to that schedule, introducing supplementary foods only after the initial six-month period, and she'll continue to breastfeed Adia until she is two.

"I did not do many things [before taking the class]," Tohomina said through a translator. "But after learning, I am keeping things clean and hygienic to prevent diseases, and cooking nutritious foods to keep me and my family healthy."

Source: Bread for the World 2013 Hunger Report

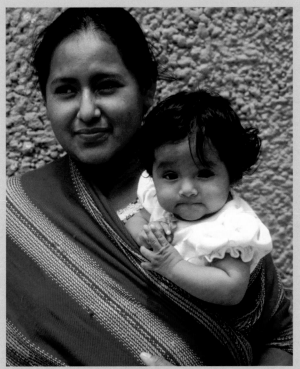

Guatemalan mother and daughter
Photo: http://www.flickr.com/photos/breadfortheworld. Source: Marsh, Molly. "Improving Nutrition Outcomes in Bangladesh." Within Reach: Global Development Goals – 2013 Hunger Report, Bread for the World Institute, pp. 14-15. Available at http://www.hungerreport.org/

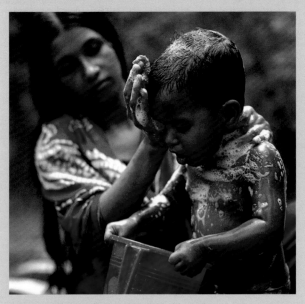

Tohomina Akter and her daughter Adia, 17 months old
Photo: http://www.flickr.com/photos/breadfortheworld. Marsh, Molly. "Improving Nutrition Outcomes in Bangladesh." Within Reach: Global Development Goals – 2013 Hunger Report, Bread for the World Institute, pp. 14-15. Available at http://www.hungerreport.org/

Further reading

UN Civil society declaration.

Bread for the World Institute. Hunger Report 2013: Within reach: Global development goals. Bread for the World Institute, 2013.

Save the Children. A life free from hunger: Tackling child malnutrition. Save the Children, 2012.

Save the Children. Food for thought, tackling child malnutrition to unlock potential and boost prosperity. Save the Children, 2013.

Action Against Hunger. Aid for nutrition: Mobilizing innovative financing for the fight against undernutrition. Action Against Hunger, 2013.

1 *http://www.bread.org/event/gathering-2011/international-meeting/*

2 *http://www.bread.org/event/gathering-2011/international-meeting/pdf/meeting-summary-report.pdf*

3 *Asma Lateef. "The Role and Capacity of Civil Society Organizations in Responding to the Economic and Food Price Crises", in IOM (Institute of Medicine). 2010. Mitigating the Nutritional Impacts of the Global Food Price Crisis: Workshop Summary, Washington , DC: The National Academies Press.*

4 *www.bread.org/meeting*

5 *http://scalingupnutrition.org/wp-content/uploads/2012/10/SUN-MP-REPORT_EN.pdf p.19*

6 *http://www.postzambia.com/post-read_article.php?articleId=29815; additional media stories include: http://www.qfmzambia.com/news_story.php?idx=11770&gone=11771&v1; http://zambiadailynation.com/2013/03/08/empower-women-to-end-poverty-cso-sun/*

7 *http://www.qfmzambia.com/blog_details.php?idx=11494*

8 *http://scalingupnutrition.org/sun-countries/tanzania/progress-impact/bringing-people-together/civil-society*

9 *World Bank (February 29, 2012), New Estimates Reveal Drop in Extreme Poverty 2005-2010, Washington, DC.*

10 *Charles Kenny and Andy Sumner (2011), "More Money or More Development: What Have the MDGs Achieved." CGD Working Paper 278. Washington, DC: Center for Global Development.*

11 *Kenny and Casabonne (2008), "The Best Things in Life are Nearly Free: Technology, Ideas, and Global Quality of Life," Center for Global Development.*

12 *See Charles Kenny and Andy Sumner (2011).*

13 *http://thousanddays.org/wp-content/uploads/2012/05/WHO-Targets-Policy-Brief.pdf*

14 *http://documents.worldbank.org/curated/en/2013/02/17428493/nutrition-post-2015-development-agenda-report-expert-consultation*

15 *United Nations (2013), A New Global Partnership: Eradicate Poverty and Transform Economies Through Sustainable Development. The Report of the High-Level Panel of Eminent Persons on the Post-2015 Development Agenda.*

16 *HLP Report, pp. 29-30*

My personal view

Asma Lateef
Director, Bread for the World Institute
Washington DC, USA

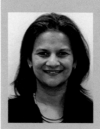

Over the past four years, the nutrition landscape has been completely transformed. New knowledge, increased attention to hunger and food insecurity as a result of the food price crisis, and effective collaboration across stakeholders have led to the rise of the SUN Movement.

Civil society played an important role in making the case for action on nutrition. As a result of the governments of the United Kingdom and Brazil and Children's Investment Fund Foundation's Nutrition for Growth High Level Meeting in London on June 8, 2013, we now have impressive new financial and nutrition outcome commitments from donors, international organizations, the private sector and non-governmental organizations.

One could be forgiven for thinking that the work is done! Now is not the time for complacency, however. The commitments have to be fulfilled. More importantly, resources and policies must result in dramatic reductions in the number of stunted children.

In order to ensure sustained political commitment, civil society needs to speak with unified, clear messages about the importance of nutrition in the post-2015 development goals. Communicating how fundamental good nutrition in the pregnancy and early childhood is to ending extreme poverty must be part of advocacy efforts in the near future.

There will be many interests and issues that will be under consideration. Countries that are taking steps to scale up nutrition are uniquely placed to make the case for including a nutrition goal, indicators and targets. Civil society can advocate for them to do just that.

Chapter Thirteen

The Evolving World of Nutrition

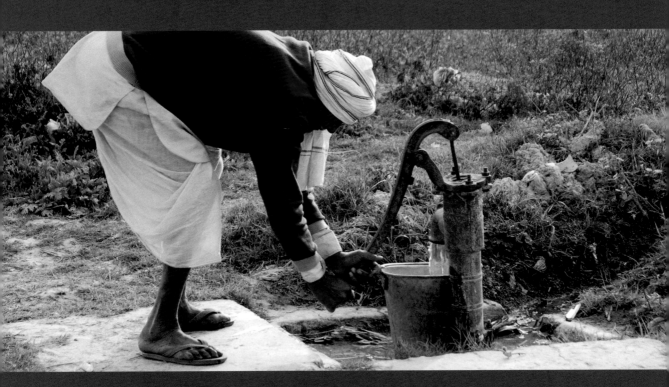

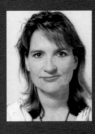

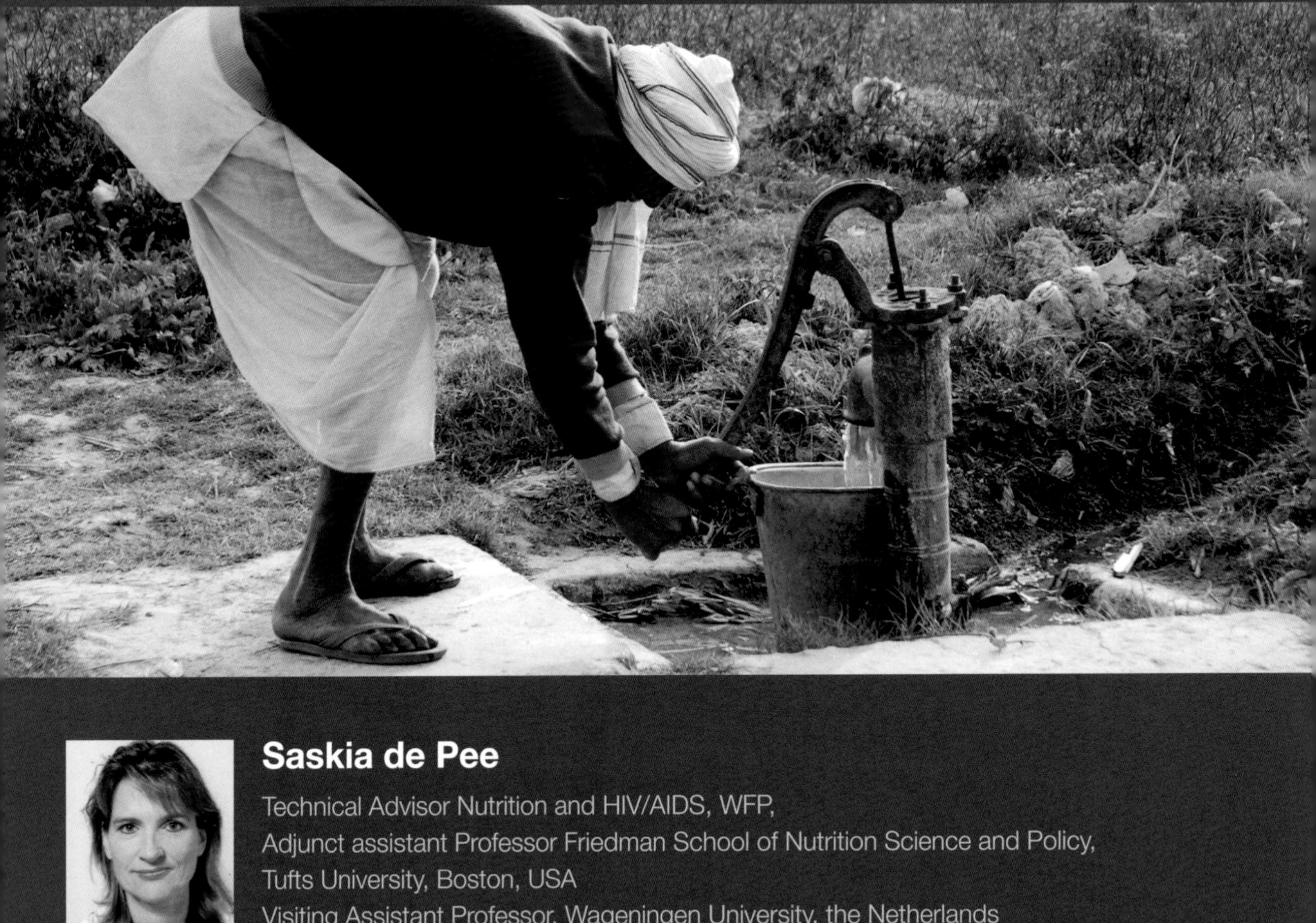

Saskia de Pee

Technical Advisor Nutrition and HIV/AIDS, WFP,
Adjunct assistant Professor Friedman School of Nutrition Science and Policy,
Tufts University, Boston, USA
Visiting Assistant Professor, Wageningen University, the Netherlands

"He who has health has hope, and he who has hope has everything."

Arabian Proverb

Key messages

- Almost everyone plays a role in nutrition through taking care of their own diet and health, as well as through involvement in the food system in one way or another.

- Nutrition is multi-disciplinary, ranging from agriculture to medicine to behavioral science and economics.

- Throughout the 20th century, knowledge and approaches for addressing malnutrition developed within the respective disciplines, but there was limited cross-disciplinary coordination, even with other players in the food and health systems.

- Understanding the forms and consequences of undernutrition, being able to cost the economic impact of undernutrition, and having examples of what is required and what works to prevent undernutrition, including good governance, has generated the strong momentum behind nutrition that exists today.

Nutrition is everybody's business

Everyone deals with nutrition – individuals who are looking after their own diet and health; mothers and fathers who are caring for their families; farmers who grow food for themselves and others; medical doctors, teachers, sports coaches and others who support people in understanding the importance of health and nutrition; food processors who produce, preserve, package and distribute foods; and community leaders, politicians and business owners, who impact other people's ability to access an affordable, healthy and nutritious diet. Food systems around the world are diverse, increasingly industrial, commercial and global, and many of us play an active role in shaping them.

However, while we affect our own and other people's nutrition every day, directly or indirectly, there are many different ways in which nutrition and health are understood, and our ability and decisions to actively influence them, either by ourselves or by seeking assistance from others, ranges widely. Furthermore, as the preceding chapters discuss, many factors that impact on the health and nutrition of individuals and populations are beyond the direct influence of the individual, as these are determined by their environment and circumstances.

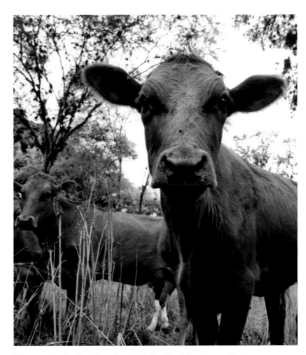

Silvopastoral cultivation, in which livestock live in wooded areas
Source: CIAT

171 Early discoveries in nutrition

Throughout the centuries, there has been a growing understanding of the relationship between diet and health and about how poverty and related living circumstances affect a population's health, for a substantial part through the diet.

In the late 19th and early 20th centuries, scientists in the fields of chemistry, biology and medicine started conducting animal experiments in which they supplemented basic diets consisting of carbohydrates, fat and protein, with specific foods or food components such as milk and butter to determine which components made the animals live or die. While doing so, they observed conditions in the animals that were comparable to symptoms that had been described in humans, such as in records from naval medicine in the 19th century.

Over the course of a few decades, the various vitamins were isolated and named, and their deficiency states described. For several of the deficiencies, the ultimate consequence was death. It was realized that severe deficiencies could occur without starvation, and that many people were probably affected by nutritional deficiencies. To address vitamin A deficiency, some European countries and the US introduced school milk distribution schemes (fortified with vitamin A in the case of skimmed milk) as well as encouraging, or even enforcing, consumption of butter and/or cod liver oil in the 1920s–1940s.

Vitamin	Alternative name	Discovery	Isolation	Structure	Synthesis
Vitamin A	Retinol	1909	1931	1931	1947
Provitamin A	β-Carotene	1831	1831	1930	1950
Vitamin D	Calciferol	1918	1932	1936	1959
Vitamin E	Tocopherol	1922	1936	1938	1938
Vitamin K	Phylloquinone	1929	1939	1939	1939
Vitamin B1	Thiamin	1897	1926	1936	1936
Vitamin B2	Riboflavin	1920	1933	1935	1935
Vitamin B3	Niacin	1936	1936	1937	1994
Vitamin B5	Pantothenic acid	1931	1938	1940	1940
Vitamin B6	Pyridoxine	1934	1938	1938	1939
Vitamin B7	Biotin	1931	1935	1942	1943
Vitamin B9	Folic acid	1941	1941	1946	1946
Vitamin B12	Cobalamin	1926	1948	1956	1972
Vitamin C	Ascorbic acid	1912	1928	1933	1933

From November 1944 to December 1945, 36 conscientious objectors participated in the historical Minnesota Starvation Experiment, which was designed to study the physiological and psychological effects of severe and prolonged dietary restriction and the effect of dietary rehabilitation strategies, as was a reality for many people in Europe during the Second World War. This work, led by Ancel Keys, provided key insights into nutrition, including the understanding that starvation dramatically alters personality and that nutrition directly, and predictably, affects mind as well as body.

During that first half of the 20th century, undernutrition was primarily of interest a) as a medical condition with specific symptoms characterizing specific nutrient deficiencies, and b) as a problem of lack of food resulting in starvation.

Different worlds of nutrition

Between the 1940s and 1970s, the medical field evolved dramatically, and after the Second World War, the economic development of Western Europe and North America increased access to a more nutritious diet for a large part of the population, while living circumstances such as hygiene and education continued to improve substantially. Together, these developments resulted in lower child mortality, increased life expectancy, and a marked reduction of nutrient deficiency diseases (e.g rickets and night blindness).

With these developments, the momentum behind nutrition in Europe and North America from the early part of the 20th century was not sustained, as undernutrition was not perceived to be much of a problem anymore. The attention for the role of nutrition in health continued in developing countries and among international agencies, and regained strength globally when case reports and survey data on health and nutrition started to be reported from more and more developing countries from the early 1970s.

In the period following the Second World War, most of the attention regarding diet and food was focused on ensuring that there would be enough food for the growing world population, and on making sure that protein deficiency was prevented or treated (see the chapter in this volume by Victoria Quinn on the 'protein fiasco'). This meant that agriculture was largely focused on the production of cereals (green revolution, increase of scale) to ensure that caloric requirements were met, and on cash crops for income.

The signs of undernutrition from developing countries that drew attention from professionals in the biomedical field were particularly those related to micronutrient deficiencies, which could be solved by a medical-type intervention, such as providing supplements of vitamin A, iron, iodine and/or zinc.

Meanwhile, it was also realized that the causes of nutrition problems were rooted in poverty, and that, besides being related to food, they were also related to water, hygiene, sanitation and caring practices, and that approaches for addressing malnutrition therefore had to be multi-disciplinary. Due to this, social and behavioral scientists also became involved in nutrition, and there was an increasing sense that individuals and communities should be able to rely on their own resources and means, including food production, to achieve adequate nutrition.

The UNICEF Conceptual Framework of causes of malnutrition, which was developed at the time of the Iringa project in Tanzania in the early 1980s, clearly illustrated the multi-factorial causes of malnutrition and indirectly assigned a role for many disciplines for addressing malnutrition. However, for a couple of decades, there was limited focused attention on addressing malnutrition, because the comprehensiveness of the framework indicated that there were many factors involved but at the same time it was not clear which one(s) to prioritize where and who should take which action. There was also limited awareness of the consequences of not tackling the problem, and several signs of undernutrition were not yet properly understood.

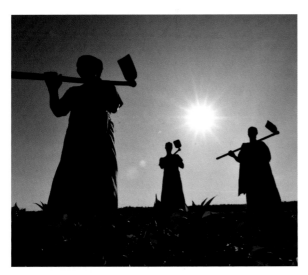

Women farmers in East Africa
Source: CIAT

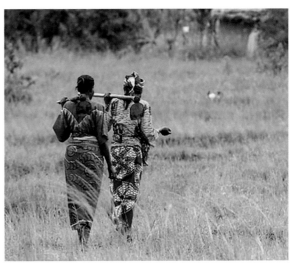

Women have a key role to play in improving the nutritional status of the world's population
Source: The Gates Foundation

Momentum for concerted action on nutrition

Fortunately, the past ten years have seen a marked increase of attention as well as momentum for action on nutrition, due to several coinciding developments:

- **Advances of our knowledge of the consequences of undernutrition**, which goes beyond the signs and symptoms of specific deficiencies on the one hand and starvation on the other, to lifetime consequences of inadequate nutrition in early life in terms of early morbidity and mortality, as well as impact on cognitive ability affecting performance in school and income-earning potential, and non-communicable diseases later in life such as cardiovascular disease and diabetes;

- **Increased understanding of the biology of malnutrition**, including the relationship between two apparently different forms of malnutrition, i.e., undernutrition and overnutrition, that are actually very much related (both include micronutrient deficiencies, both are related to poverty – the world's wealthier and well-educated people have the healthiest diet, and undernutrition in early life predisposes to overnutrition and non-communicable disease later in life);

- **Evidence of effective nutrition interventions**, including their cost-benefit ratio. Also, the Copenhagen Consensus 2012 expert panel of economists, which included four Nobel laureates, identified that the smartest ways to allocate money to respond to ten of the world's biggest challenges is by fighting malnourishment. Nobel laureate economist Vernon Smith said: "One of the most compelling investments is to get nutrients to the world's undernourished. The benefits from doing so – in terms of increased health, schooling, and productivity – are tremendous";

- **The observation that economic development and large-scale production of cheap, convenient food does not lead to better health** but instead is related to an epidemic of obesity and related non-communicable diseases, has led to people's rethinking of food systems and healthy and sustainable diets (it has become everybody's problem);

- **Increased ownership of nutrition and collaboration by a wide range of disciplines**, including biomedical, behavioral, agricultural, and economics;

- **Increased access to information** through media such as Internet and mobile-phone technology, which increases the awareness as well as the ability to act and hold politicians, companies and others accountable for their actions;

- **A more connected world** where heads of state agree on mutual goals (Millennium Development Goals, post-2015 development agenda), low-income countries evolve to become middle-income countries and grow from being the recipients of donor funding to being donors themselves, and the private sector becomes involved in solving the problems of the most vulnerable.

The first Lancet series on Maternal and Child Nutrition, which was published in 2008, summarized the magnitude and consequences of the nutrition problem, and provided evidence of a number of proven and low-cost solutions. This publication galvanized substantial action on multiple fronts, and not only the questions of 'why to address undernutrition, by doing **what**, and **where**', but also the question of '**how** to do it' received attention. Moreover, this happened at a time when it was realized that everyone has a role to play, including, for example, the private sector, which had previously been regarded by some as mainly contributing to the problem rather than building a path to the solution. It also showed convincingly that poor fetal growth or stunting in the first two years of life leads to irreversible damage, including shorter adult height, lower attained schooling, reduced adult income, and decreased offspring birth weight. This very much focused everyone's attention on the prevention of stunting and on prioritizing nutrition during the first thousand days from conception until two years of age.

Furthermore, in May 2012, the 65th World Health Assembly (WHA) endorsed six global nutrition targets to be achieved by 2025 as part of WHO's comprehensive plan on maternal, infant and young child nutrition, including reducing by 40 percent the number of children under age 5 who are stunted from 171 million in 2010 to 100 million by 2025. This means that there is very broad commitment to these goals, as the WHA is the forum through which WHO is governed by its 194 member states and it is composed of health ministers from these states.

Malnutrition remains a serious impediment to the progress towards achieving the Millennium Development Goals. Yet many of the nutrition challenges that have persisted for decades can be resolved within our generation.

Recognizing that accelerated global action is needed to address the pervasive and corrosive problem of malnutrition, the World Health Organization (WHO) recently identified a set of global targets designed to reduce the unacceptably high burdens of disease and death caused by poor nutrition, particularly during the critical 1,000 days between a woman's pregnancy and a child's second birthday.* By aligning the glocal community behind six targets aimed at improving the nutritional status of mothers, infants and young children and committing to a decade of investement to expand nutrition interventions, we can prevent the deaths of one million children per year and help to build the foundations for healthier and more prosperous societies.

GLOBAL TARGET 1

By 2025, reduce by 40% the number of children under age 5 who are stunted.

Problem:
Stunting is the irreversible result of chronic nutritional deprivation during the most critical phase of child development - the 1,000 days between a woman's pregnancy and her child's 2nd birthday. Stunted children have weaker immune systems making them more likely to die from common illnesses and disease, and suffer from impaired brain development making them less able to learn in school and earn a good living as an adult.

Results:
A reduction in the number of stunted children from 171 million in 2010 to approximately 100 million.

GLOBAL TARGET 2

By 2025, achieve a 50% reduction in anemia in women of reproductive age.

Problem:
Anemia in women increases the risk of dying during childbirth and increases the risk of babies being born with low birth weight. Iron deficiency anemia affects 1/3 of all women of reproductive age throughout the world.

Results:
A reduction in the number of anemic, non-pregnant women from 468 million to approximately 230 million.

GLOBAL TARGET 3

By 2025, achieve a 30% reduction of the number of infants born with low birth weight.

Problem:
An infant's weight at birth is a strong indicator of his or her chances for survival, growth, and long-term health and development. In the developing world, low birth weight stems primarily from poor maternal nutritional status before conception, maternal short stature due mostly to undernutrition and infections during childhood and poor nutrition during pregnancy.

Results:
3.9% relative reduction in the number of infants born with low birth weight per year.

GLOBAL TARGET 4

By 2025, ensure that there is no increase in the number of children who are overweight.

Problem:
Obese children are likely to grow into obese adults, have an increased risk of diabetes and liver disease, and have poorer economic prospects later in life.

Results:
The number of overweight children under age 5 would not increase from current levels of 43 million to forecasted levels of approximately 70 million.

GLOBAL TARGET 5

By 2025, increase to at least 50% the rate of exclusive breastfeeding in the first six months.

Problem:
A non-breastfed child is 14 times more likely to die in their first six months of life than a child who is exclusively breastfed. Though breastfeeding is the single most effective nutrition intervention for saving lives, global breastfeeding rates have stagnated or dropped in most regions of the world to an estimated 37%.

Results:
2.3% relative increase per year would lead to approximately 10 million more children per year being exclusively breastfed until six months of age.

GLOBAL TARGET 6

By 2025, reduce and maintain childhood wasting to less than 5%

Problem:
Commonly used to indicate the severity of a famine of food crisis, wasting is the result of grave disease and/or deprivation of nutritious food at a specific point in time and is seen as an early warning for future increases in chronic undernutrition. The proportion of childhood wasting rose in the second half of the last decade, likely as a consequence of the dramatic spikes in food prices.

Results:
Current global prevalence of wasting of 8.6% should be reduced to less than 5% by 2025 and maintained below such levels.

*These targets were endorsed by the 65th World Health Assembly in May 2012 as part of WHO's comprehensive plan on maternal, infant and young child nutrition. Sources: Black, R. et al "Maternal and Child Undernutrition" The Lancet, January 2008; Save the Children "The Child Development Index 2012"; UNICEF, "Committing to Child Survival: A Promise Renewed" Progress Report 2012.

175

The second Lancet series of 2013 has reaffirmed the findings of the first series and particularly emphasizes the importance of adequate nutrition for pregnant and lactating women as well as for adolescent girls (before they become pregnant). It also highlights the potential for nutrition-sensitive fields and programming to contribute to preventing undernutrition and/or deliver some nutrition-specific interventions.

The current momentum in nutrition is particularly coordinated through the SUN (Scaling Up Nutrition) Movement, to which more than 40 countries have now committed themselves. They have committed to implementing nutrition-specific and nutrition-sensitive action, and have joined a movement that is coordinated by a special representative to the UN Secretary-General and has been endorsed by more than 100 organizations.

Conclusion

The world of nutrition has evolved substantially over the last century and a half, reaching a high level of knowledge, convergence and momentum, especially during the past ten years. This should result in more sustainable and nutritious diets and in better health and life chances for children being born in the next few decades.

My personal view

Saskia de Pee
Technical Advisor Nutrition and HIV/AIDS, WFP
Adjunct assistant Professor Friedman School of Nutrition Science and Policy, Tufts University, Boston.
Visiting Assistant Professor, Wageningen University, the Netherlands

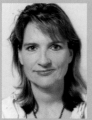

Having worked in the field of nutrition for almost 20 years, I find this time very exciting because of the great momentum to improve nutrition and health worldwide and the increased understanding and commitment among a very wide range of stakeholders and experts.

The involvement of so many is essential, and while everyone should focus on what they are good at, there is a great deal of cross-disciplinary work to be done in a target-oriented manner.

It is important to develop context-specific solutions based on the global body of knowledge and expertise, and to monitor, evaluate and share these experiences using the information and communication technology available today.

Further reading

Bloem MW, de Pee S, Semba RD. How much do data influence programs for health and nutrition? Experiences from Health and Nutrition Surveillance Systems. In: Semba RD, Bloem MW (eds). Nutrition and Health in Developing Countries (2nd ed). Totowa, NY: Humana Press, 2008.

Copenhagen Consensus. http://www.copenhagenconsensus.com/projects/copenhagenconsensus-2012/outcome

Food and Agriculture Organization. The State of Food and Agriculture. Rome: FAO, 2013.

Kalm LM, Semba RD. They starved so that others be better fed: Remembering Ancel Keys and the Minnesota Experiment. J Nutr 2005;135:1347–1352.

Sight and Life. Micronutrients, macro-impact: The story of vitamins and a hungry world. Basel, Switzerland: Sight and Life, 2012.

The SUN Movement website: www.scalingupnutrition.org

Table 1: Progress in Micronutrient Science and Policy

1975	Formation of International Vitamin A Consultative Group (IVACG)
1991	Ending Hidden Hunger: The Montreal Micronutrient Conference, Montreal, Canada
1992	Helen Keller International Bellagio Meeting on Vitamin A Deficiency and Childhood Mortality
2002	UN General Assembly special session on children
	Creation of GAIN (Global Alliance for Improved Nutrition)
2006	Creation of Micronutrient Forum
2007	World Bank report Repositioning Nutrition as Central to Development
2008	Lancet Series, Maternal and Child Undernutrition
	Copenhagen Consensus places micronutrients center stage
	World Economy Forum formed the Global Agenda Council (GAC) on Food Security
2009	Castel Gandolfo Declaration
	Private Sector Declaration and United Call to Action on Vitamins and Mineral Deficiencies during Micronutrient Forum, Beijing
	Creation of Amsterdam Initiative for Malnutrition (AIM)
	Obama administration signals its commitment to addressing hunger
	International Congress on Nutrition in Bangkok – Nutrition Security for All
	G8's $20 billion commitment on Food Security and Nutrition
	Scaling Up Nutrition (SUN): A Framework for Action – up-scaling of 13 highly cost-effective interventions
2010	G20 pledge additional $5.0 billion over the next five years towards achieving MDGs 4&5
	African Union summit places safe motherhood and child health high on Africa's agenda
	SUN Framework and Roadmap launched
	Feed the Future (FTF), the new US government global hunger and food security initiative, is launched
	The Global Strategy for Women's and Children's Health launched by UN Secretary-General
	UN Secretary-General includes nutrition security and the importance of nutrition at the MDG summit
	Nutrition included in the 2010 MDG outcome document
	1,000 Days Partnership: Change a Life, Change the Future launched by Hillary Rodham-Clinton, the United States Secretary of State, and Irish Minister of Foreign affairs, Micheál Martin
	African First Ladies sign a call for action to put nutrition at the heart of development.
2011	High-level event on Scaling Up Nutrition at UN Headquarters, New York (September)
2012	Copenhagen Consensus – bundled nutrition interventions ranked highest
	Hunger Summit at Olympic Games, London
2013	Hidden Hunger Conference, Hohenheim, Germany
	Launch of Lancet Series on Maternal and Child Nutrition
	Nutrition for Growth meeting, London - $4.1 billion new funding for nutrition-specific actions and $19 billion for nutrition-sensitive activities
	International Congress on Nutrition in Granada – Joining Cultures Through Nutrition
	Report of the High-Level Panel of Eminent Persons on the Post-2015 Development Agenda

Source: Amended after Micronutrients, Macro-Impact: The story of vitamins and a hungry world, Sight and Life, 2012. Copyright Sight and Life.

177 **Table 1: Important Milestones in Nutrition Policy Development**

Year	Organization	Purpose	Goals	Achieved in Moving the Agenda Forward
2002	The International Vitamin A Consultative Group (IVACG) Annecy Accord	Leading the campaign against vitamin A deficiency disorders (VADD)	- Provide a forum to exchange new ideas, to discuss research findings and their policy implications, and share experiences with program interventions. - Provide technical guidance through state-of-the-art publications on VADD. - Collaborate with international organizations in developing and establishing policy guidelines for diagnosis, treatment, and prevention of VADD.	Comprehensive recommendations for the assessment and control of vitamin A deficiency (VAD) were rigorously reviewed and revised by a working group and presented for discussion at the XX International Vitamin A Consultative Group meeting in Hanoi, Vietnam.
2007	The World Bank; Report on Repositioning Nutrition as Central to Development	Provide a global framework for action and to complement the similar analyses undertaken by the World Bank's regional units for Africa and South Asia.	- Reinvigorate dialogue regarding what to do about malnutrition; - Encourage the development community to reevaluate the priority it gives nutrition; - Facilitate an agreement on new ways for stakeholders to work together; - Scale up proven interventions for tackling malnutrition.	This report highlighted the burden of malnutrition and importance of addressing it, thereby justifying the increased funding for nutrition from the World Bank.
2008	Lancet Series; Maternal and Child Undernutrition	Given that that nutrition is a major risk factor for disease, the Lancet series sought to gather scientific evidence about the importance of maternal and child nutrition and aimed to fill this gap in global public health and policy action.	- Catalogue the long-term effects of undernutrition; - Identify proven interventions to reduce undernutrition; - Call for national and international action to improve nutrition for mothers and children.	Provided objective evidence that there are effective interventions to reduce stunting and micronutrient deficiencies and that improved governance is desperately needed to scale up nutrition interventions, monitor and evaluate those plans, and implement laws to enhance the rights of women and children.
2008	Copenhagen Consensus	To set priorities among a series of proposals for confronting the following global challenges: Air Pollution, Conflicts, Diseases, Education, Global Warming, Malnutrition and Hunger, Sanitation and Water, Subsidies and Trade Barriers, Terrorism, Women and Development.	The panel was asked to address the ten challenges by considering the question, "What would be the best ways of advancing global welfare, and particularly the welfare of the developing countries, illustrated by supposing that an additional $75 billion of resources were at their disposal over a four year initial period?"	Among all the worlds challenges identified at Copenhagen, the panel ranked malnutrition very highly, given the tremendously high benefits compared to costs. The expert panel ranked fighting malnutrition as follows, providing tremendous clout to our cause: 1. Micronutrient supplements for children (vitamin A and zinc); 3. Micronutrient fortification (iron and salt iodization); 5. Biofortification; 6. Deworming and other nutrition programs at school; 9. Community-based nutrition promotion.

Year	Organization	Purpose	Goals	Achieved in Moving the Agenda Forward
2010	SUN: A Framework for Action	Labeled as the 'forgotten' Millennium Development Goal, the primary objective of the SUN Framework is to catalyze actions to move undernutrition toward the center stage of international political and economic discourse.	The policy brief hopes to provide both the following: - An outline of the emerging framework of key considerations and priorities for action to address undernutrition; - Mobilize support for increased investment in nutrition interventions.	The SUN brief concluded that the MDGs cannot be achieved without urgent attention to nutrition. SUN is a call to action for increasing high impact interventions that address undernutrition, with more than 100 organizations having endorsed the Framework to date.
2010	A Road Map for Scaling up Nutrition	Provides the principles and direction for increased support for countries as they scale up efforts to tackle undernutrition across a range of sectors. It encourages multi-stakeholder platforms that promote synergized actions and simplify coordination of support.	To serve as a resource for countries wanting to include nutrition within the context of nutrition-focused development policies	Galvanizing countries to take nutrition seriously and include it in their development agenda.
2013	Lancet Series 2	An update of issues dealt with in Lancet 1 (2008)	Re-evaluation of the problems of maternal and child undernutriiton and also examination of the growing problems of overweight and obesity and their consequences in low- and middle-income countries	Its aim is to offer evidence-based consensus recommendations on what to do about the continuing problem of undernutrition. Particular attention is paid to costing actions of direct nutrition interventions in the context of nutrition-sensitive interventions.

Source: Amended after Micronutrients, Macro-Impact: The story of vitamins and a hungry world, Sight and Life, 2012. Copyright Sight and Life.

179 List of key organizations

Centers for Disease Control and Prevention (CDC)

Health Protection – Health Equity

Founded: 1946

Headquarters: Atlanta, GA, USA

Website: www.cdc.gov

Collaborating to create the expertise, information, and tools that people and communities need to protect their health – through health promotion, prevention of disease, injury and disability, and preparedness for new health threats.

Canadian International Development Agency (CIDA)

Founded: 1968

Headquarters: Gatineau, Quebec, Canada

Website: www.acdi-cida.gc.ca/home

Leads Canada's international efforts to help people living in poverty.

UK Department for International Development (DfID)

UK Government Department responsible for promoting development and the reduction of poverty

Founded: 1997

Headquarters: London and East Kilbride, Glasgow, UK

Website: www.DfID.gov.uk

DfID's mission is to eliminate global poverty by making a greater impact on achieving the Millennium Development Goals.

Food and Agriculture Organization of the United Nations (FAO)

For a world without hunger

Founded: 1945

Headquarters: Rome, Italy

Website: www.fao.org

Achieving food security for all is at the heart of FAO's efforts – to make sure people have regular access to enough high-quality food to lead active, healthy lives

GAIN (Global Alliance for Improved Nutrition)

Founded: 2002

Headquarters: Geneva, Switzerland

Website: www.gainhealth.org

GAIN is committed to accomplishing the global health goals which are related to its vision of a world without malnutrition.

Bill and Melinda Gates Foundation (Gates Foundation)

All lives have equal value

Founded: 1994

Headquarters: Seattle, Washington, USA

Website: www.gatesfoundation.org

To increase opportunity and equity for those most in need.

Helen Keller International (HKI)

HKI is a non-profit organization dedicated to preventing blindness and reducing malnutrition worldwide

Founded: 1915

Headquarters: New York City, NY, USA

Website: www.hki.org

HKI's mission is to save the sight and lives of the most vulnerable and disadvantaged. It combats the causes and consequences of blindness and malnutrition by establishing programs based on evidence and research in vision, health and nutrition.

International Food Policy Research Institute (IFPRI)

Sustainable solutions for ending hunger and poverty

Founded: 1975

Headquarters: Washington, DC, USA

Website: www.ifpri.org

To provide policy solutions that reduce poverty and end hunger and malnutrition.

International Fund for Agricultural Development (IFAD)

Founded: 1977

Headquarters: Rome, Italy

Website: www.ifad.org

The goal of the IFAD is to enable poor rural people to improve their food and nutrition security, increase their incomes and strengthen their resilience. IFAD also acts as an advocate for poor rural women and men. The multilateral orientation provides a strong global platform for discussing rural policy issues and increasing awareness of why investment in agriculture and rural development is critical to reducing poverty and improving global food security.

Micronutrient Initiative (MI)

Solutions for hidden hunger

Founded: 1997

Headquarters: Ottawa, Canada

Website: www.micronutrient.org

To develop, implement and monitor innovative, cost-effective and sustainable solutions for hidden hunger, in partnership with others.

Program for Appropriate Technology in Health (PATH)

A catalyst for global health

Founded: 1977

Headquarters: Seattle, Washington, USA

Website: www.path.org

PATH's mission is to improve the health of people around the world by advancing technologies, strengthening systems, and encouraging healthy behaviors.

United Nations International Fund (UNICEF)

'Unite for Children'

Founded: 1946

Headquarters: New York, NY, USA

Website: www.unicef.org

UNICEF is mandated by the United Nations General Assembly to advocate for the protection of children's rights, to help meet their basic needs and to expand their opportunities to reach their full potential.

United Nations World Food Program (WFP)

Fighting Hunger Worldwide

Founded: 1963

Headquarters: Rome, Italy

Website: www.wfp.org

WFP is the food-assistance agency of the United Nations system. Food assistance is one of the many instruments that can help to promote food security, which is defined as access of all people at all times to the food needed for an active and healthy life. The policies governing the use of WFP food assistance must be oriented towards the objective of eradicating hunger and poverty. Recently, WFP moved its focus from food aid to food assistance, using different modalities to improve food security and nutrition of their beneficiaries.

United States Agency for International Development (USAID)

Founded: 1961

Headquarters: Washington, DC, USA

Website: www.usaid.gov

The US Agency for International Development (USAID) is an independent agency that provides economic, development and humanitarian assistance around the world in support of the foreign policy goals of the United States.

World Health Organization (WHO)

'Working for Health'

Founded: 1948

Headquarters: Geneva, Switzerland

Website: www.who.int

WHO is the directing and coordinating authority for health within the United Nations system. It is responsible for providing leadership on global health matters, shaping the health research agenda, setting norms and standards, articulating evidence-based policy options, providing technical support to countries and monitoring and assessing health trends. In the 21st century, health is a shared responsibility, involving equitable access to essential care and collective defense against transnational threats.

The World Bank (World Bank)

Working for a world free of poverty

Founded: 1944

Headquarters: Washington, DC, USA

Website: www.worldbank.org

To fight poverty with passion and professionalism for lasting results. To help people help themselves and their environment by providing resources, sharing knowledge, building capacity and forging partnerships in the public and private sectors.

World Vision International

Founded: 1950

Headquarters: Monrovia, USA

Website: www.wvi.org

World Vision is a global Christian relief, development and advocacy organization dedicated to working with children, families and communities to overcome poverty and injustice. World Vision serves all people, regardless of religion, race, ethnicity, or gender.

Afterword:
Now is the Time

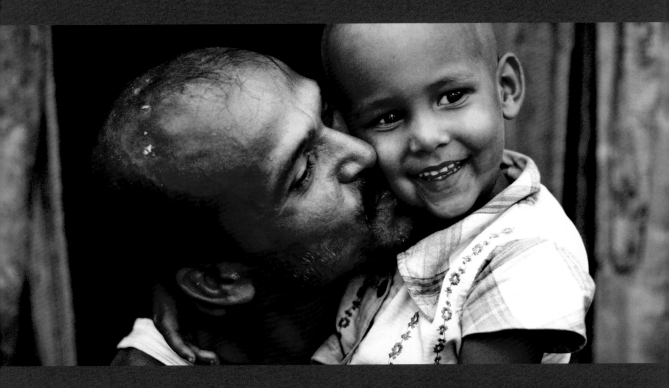

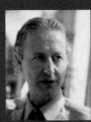

Patrick Webb

Dean for Academic Affairs,
Friedman School of Nutrition Science and Policy,
Tufts University, Boston, USA

Does the world really need this book? Do the shelves of analysts and policy-makers need the weight of yet another compendium of ideas, statistics and rhetoric?

The answer, perhaps surprisingly, is yes. Such a book is needed now, more than ever, because it reflects the rapid convergence of opinion around priority problems and likely pathways towards solutions.

The 2008 Lancet Series on Maternal and Child Undernutrition highlighted what was then called the "fragmented and dysfunctional" state of the international nutrition system.[1] That "the system is broken" became an oft-repeated mantra of the late 2000s, a signal that perhaps the biggest challenges to be faced came from within. Progress towards common purpose in nutrition had long been plagued by poorly articulated technical definitions, nutrient-centric debates, and competing institutional mandates. As a result, donor funding dedicated to nutrition was scarce, national governments chose to focus on other priorities offering more obvious gain, and science paid more attention to demonstrating the efficacy of narrowly defined interventions than to explaining how to make policies and programs work.

The calls have been heard

A mere half decade later, things are starting to look different. Calls for more resources, for greater political prioritization, and for more effective implementation of nutrition actions are being heeded. There is still a long way to go, no doubt, but the calls are being heard in the grand halls of governance, as in the corridors of academia and under the shade trees of civil society. Commitment to change is growing rapidly among developing-country politicians, donor funding has risen, scientists are sheathing their swords, and even private industry is sometimes invited to the table of global debate.

The 2013 Lancet series[2] update on maternal and child nutrition only used the term "dysfunctional" once, and then to describe how things were, not how they have become. Instead, the new series focused on the importance of accelerating evidence-based actions at scale, the essential complementarity offered by nutrition-sensitive programming that address underlying determinants, and on the need to sustain all initiatives (politically as well as financially) by shaping effective policy processes.

These changes in the tone of global discourse, linked to widespread adoption of a common lens through which to scrutinize what we do and how, represent a pivotal moment in humanity's recurring war on want. There is a sense running throughout this book that the attainment of sound nutrition for all people everywhere is no longer a fantastical dream, but a genuine possibility.

It is imperative that we act

If accepted as truly possible, it is imperative that we act in ways that make it so. The foregoing chapters articulate that great progress has recently been made in reducing prevalence rates of stunting; but 165 million children are still affected.[3] Wasting has fallen globally, but only slowly and not much in Africa. Most micronutrient deficiencies remain poorly measured and hard to uncouple from the poor diets and poor health that continue to blight more than a billion people. Obesity and chronic non-communicable diseases are spreading rapidly – now manifest as much in developing, as in industrialized, countries. Thus, the world cannot afford to treat one problem at a time. Improving nutrition in all of its forms is a massive unfinished social, economic, political and humanitarian agenda. Progress is still not fast enough or far-reaching enough to prevent the deaths and blighted lives of many hundreds of millions of people, including those still to be born in the coming decade. It has to be accelerated, made fully inclusive, and sustained.

None of which is easy. The task at hand is complex, so the solutions are anything but simple. Evidence-supported actions are needed on a wide scale to address the very specific requirements of adolescent girls, pregnant women, mothers and their infants, and children as they grow and develop into productive adults. Some actions must be pursued with universal coverage, but others must be targeted at the most urgent cases first. Some must prevent, protect and promote, but other actions that save and treat and make whole again are equally relevant to the common goal. Appropriate policies are needed to enhance the nutritional resiliency of individuals as well as of entire populations. Disasters that all too often erode past gains must be anticipated so that effective responses can be prosecuted with necessary vigor. And carefully designed activities supportive of agricultural and income growth, social protection, quality education and health represent essential contributions to the solution set. A critical component of all of the above is the generation of high-quality empirical evidence of what works best in what context.

This book captures the fact that there has not been a time in recent decades when so many people agreed on what needs to be done or why. The momentum has to be maintained. The next decade of the 21st century should be focused squarely on a global effort to get it done well, while documenting how. Unless coherent, cost-effective actions with measurable impacts quickly emerge from the current cresting wave of goodwill toward nutrition, the wait for another may be far too long. Now is the time.

References

1. Morris S, B Cogill, R Uauy, for the Maternal and Child Undernutrition Study Group. Effective international action against undernutrition: why has it proven so difficult and what can be done to accelerate progress? Lancet 2008;371;608–21.

2. The Lancet. Maternal and Child Nutrition. Special Series of four papers and related Commentaries. June 6, 2013. http://www.thelancet.com/series maternal-and-child-nutrition.

3. UNICEF. Improving Child Nutrition: The achievable imperative for global progress. New York:UNICEF, 2013.

Profiles of Contributors and Editorial Board members

I. Contributors

1. Tom Arnold

2. Hans Konrad Biesalski

3. Martin Bloem

4. Joachim von Braun

5. Alan Dangour

6. Stuart Gillespie

7. John Hoddinott

8. Eileen Kennedy

9. Alain Labrique

10. Asma Lateef

11. Marguerite B Lucea

12. Victoria Quinn

13. Marie Ruel

14. Werner Schultink

15. Patrick Webb

II. Editorial Board members

1. Manfred Eggersdorfer

2. Klaus Kraemer

3. Marie Ruel

4. Marc Van Ameringen

5. Hans Konrad Biesalski

6. Martin Bloem

7. Junshi Chen

8. Asma Lateef

9. Venkatesh Mannar

Marc Van Ameringen

Current title:

Executive Director of Global Alliance for Improved Nutrition (GAIN), Geneva, Switzerland

Qualification:

MA in Political Science

Focus:

Leadership roles for nonprofit organizations in the area of nutrition and development.

Biography:

A Canadian national, Marc Van Ameringen has spent more than twenty years working in the field of international development. He is the Executive Director of the Global Alliance for Improved Nutrition (GAIN), which supports programs aimed at reducing malnutrition with a focus on micronutrient deficiencies.

Under his leadership, GAIN has become a major alliance of business, governments and international organizations that is implementing at scale nutrition programs in more than 30 countries. These innovative market-driven programs are improving the lives of over nearly 800 million people, of which more than half are women and children.

Prior to joining GAIN in December 2004, Marc was Vice President of the Canada-based Micronutrient Initiative (MI), where he was responsible for coordination, planning and management of MI programs. Before this, he was Special Advisor to the G8 Summit within the Canadian Government's Department of Foreign Affairs and International Trade, assisting the G8 in responding to the New Partnership for Africa's Development (NEPAD) initiative.

From 1992 to 2002, Marc was a Director based in Africa for the International Development Research Centre (IDRC), responsible for a number of large development programs across Africa. He played an important role in assisting South Africa and other countries in Southern Africa in their reconstruction and development. Prior to moving to Africa, he held various senior positions in Canada for IDRC and other organizations.

Marc has served as a Board Member and Trustee of many different development organizations and has published a number of books on development in Africa. In 2008, he was appointed a Member of the Institute of Medicine's Committee on U.S. Commitment to Global Health. In 2009, he was nominated Vice Chair of the World Economic Forum's Global Agenda Council on Nutrition.

Tom Arnold

Current title:

Chairman of the Convention on the Irish Constitution

Qualification:

MA in Business Administration, Catholic University of Louvain

MA in Strategic Management, Trinity College, Dublin

BA in Agricultural Economics, University College, Dublin

Focus:

Governmental and charity organizations in Ireland and internationally; management, policy development and administration.

Biography:

Mr Arnold was CEO of Concern Worldwide from 2001 until February 2013. Concern Worldwide is Ireland's largest humanitarian organization and has a growing presence in the United Kingdom and the USA. Its work focuses on helping the most vulnerable people in the world's poorest countries.

Innovation and influence

During his tenure as CEO, Mr Arnold led Concern through a period of growth in budget, operations, innovation and influence.

Additional engagements include:

- Member of the Lead Group of the Scaling Up Nutrition (SUN) Movement, 2012 - present

- Member of the Consortium Board for International Agricultural Research (CGIAR), 2010-2012

- Member of the Consortium Board of the Consultative Group for International Agricultural Research since 2009

- Member of the International Food Policy Research Institute's 2020 Advisory Board since 2006

- Chair of the Irish Times Trust and Member of the Irish Times Board

- Chair of European Food Security Group, a network of European NGOs, from 2005-2010

- Member of Irish government's Commission on Taxation from 2005-2009

- Member of Advisory Board for the UN's Central Emergency Response Fund 2006-2009

- Member of Irish government's Hunger Task Force 2007-2008

- Member of UN Millennium Project's Hunger Task Force 2003-2005

Victoria Quinn

Current title:

Senior Vice President of Programs, Helen Keller International, New York, USA

Adjunct Associate Professor, Friedman School of Nutrition Science and Policy, Boston, USA

Qualification:

PhD in nutrition planning and policy from Wageningen University, Wageningen, the Netherlands

Focus:

Nutrition policy, planning and surveillance, infant and young child feeding, micronutrients and women's nutrition

Biography:

Dr Quinn joined Helen Keller International in 2006 as Senior Vice President of Programs, and is based in Washington, DC. She has more than 30 years of experience in Africa, Asia, and Latin America, designing and managing complex and large-scale nutrition and maternal child health country and regional programs, including those involving agriculture and nutrition.

Dr Quinn's areas of expertise include nutrition policy and surveillance, infant and young child feeding, micronutrients and women's nutrition. She received her Bachelor's and Master's in nutrition from UC Berkeley and Cornell University, respectively, and her Doctorate from Wageningen University in the Netherlands.

From 1982–1991, she served as the Regional Coordinator of Cornell University's collaborative program with UNICEF in Eastern and Southern Africa supporting country initiatives in nutritional surveillance and food and nutrition policy. Thereafter, she worked as a consultant for UNICEF, WHO, WFP, the World Bank and the Dutch government on a variety of food and nutrition security issues related to Africa. From 1998–2006 Dr Quinn served as the senior technical manager for the LINKAGES Project's flagship infant and young child feeding programs in Bolivia, Ethiopia, Ghana, Madagascar and the Horn of Africa. She also co-directed AED's Center for Nutrition from 2001–2006.

In 2007, Dr Quinn was appointed Adjunct Associate Professor, at the Friedman School of Nutrition Science and Policy at Tufts University in Boston. She is currently on the Technical Advisory Groups for Tufts' Nutrition CRSP Program, Bread for the World, as well as serving as a member of the International Advisory Panel for GAIN's Access to Nutrition Index study. Since 2007 she has chaired the sub-working Group on 'Integrating Breastfeeding with the Appropriate Marketing of Complementary Foods' under the Maternal, Infant and Young Child Nutrition Working Group. Dr Quinn has also been an active member of the Scaling Up Nutrition Civil Society network since its inception.

Further information:

http://www.hki.org/about-us/our-organization/senior-leadership/

Marie Ruel

Current title:

Director, Poverty, Health and Nutrition Division, International Food Policy Research Institute (IFPRI), Washington DC, USA

Qualification:

PhD in International Nutrition from Cornell University, Ithaca, USA

Focus:

Poverty and maternal and child malnutrition in developing countries; related policies and programs

Biography:

Dr Ruel was appointed Director of IFPRI's Poverty, Health and Nutrition Division Food in 2004. From 1996 to 2004, she served as (senior) research fellow in that division and successively led two large multi-country and regional programs: one on urban food security and nutrition and one on diet quality and diet changes of the poor. Prior to IFPRI, she was head of the Nutrition and Health Division at the Institute of Nutrition of Central America and Panama / Pan American Health Organization (INCAP/PAHO) in Guatemala, where she lived and worked for 6 years. Dr Ruel received her PhD in International Nutrition from Cornell University and her Master's in Health Sciences from Laval University in Canada.

Dr Ruel has worked for more than 25 years on policies and programs to alleviate poverty and malnutrition in developing countries. She has published extensively in nutrition and epidemiology journals on topics such as maternal and child nutrition, agriculture-and food-based strategies to improve diet quality and micronutrient nutrition, urban livelihoods, food security and nutrition, the development and validation of indicators of child feeding and care practices, and program evaluation. Her current research focuses on the evaluation and strengthening of a wide range of integrated, multi-sectoral development programs in the area of social protection and agriculture and at building the evidence on their role in reducing maternal and child malnutrition globally. She has served on various international expert committees, such as the National Academy of Sciences, the International Zinc in Nutrition Consultative Group, the Society for International Nutrition Research, and has recently joined the Micronutrient Forum Steering Committee. She recently led the development of a large CGIAR program on Agriculture for Improved Nutrition and Health, and is currently contributing to its successful implementation.

Further information:

http://www.ifpri.org/staffprofile/marie-ruel

Jan Werner Schultink

Current title:

Associate Director, Nutrition Section, Programme Division, UNICEF, New York

Qualification:

PhD in Scientific Research from the Agricultural University of Wageningen, Wageningen, The Netherlands

Focus:

Development and delivery of Nutrition Programes

Biography:

Dr Schultink is the Associate Director of the Nutrition Section, Programme Division for the UNICEF Headquarters in New York. He gives guidance and advice on the global overall direction and strategies for the Nutrition programming of UNICEF, and he acts as the principal liaison on UNICEF Nutrition issues for other relevant UN agencies, NGOs and donor governments and agencies. Dr Schultink is responsible for the management of the Nutrition Section and its 16 professional staff, and he assists in fund raising.

Prior to this, Dr Schultink was the Officer in Charge of the Nutrition Section in the UNICEF Headquarters in New York, a role which he fulfilled in addition to his role as Senior Advisor of Micronutrient Programs at UNICEF Headquarters.

From 1990 to 1999, Dr Schultink acted as long-term advisor for the "Deutsche Gesellschaft für Technische Zusammenarbeit (GTZ)" in the field of human nutrition at the Regional South-East Asian Ministers of Education Organization (SEAMEO) Center for Community Nutrition, located at the University of Indonesia, Jakarta.

Dr Schultink achieved his PhD in Scientific Research in1991 from the University of Wageningen. During the writing of his thesis, Seasonal variation in nutritional status and energy requirements of rural Beninese women, Dr Schultink was placed in a rural district of the Republic of Benin, West Africa, where he carried out research according to the framework of co-operation with the Agricultural Faculty of the University of Benin.

Dr Schultink was appointed the Adjunct Associate Professor, at the Friedman School of Nutrition Science and Policy, Tufts University, Boston in May 2009. He was also the Vice-Chair of the Standing Committee on Nutrition of the United Nations System between September 2007 and Januray 2009; a board member of a Partnership for the sustainable elimination of iodine deficiency through the iodization of salt; a member of the Steering Committee of the Micronutrient Initiative, a Canadian-based NGO funded by the Canadian Government, between April 1999 and October 2001; and Secretary and Co-Chairperson of the ACC/SCN Working Group on Maternal Nutrition and Low Birth Weight between May 2000 and December 2002.

Patrick Webb

Current title:

Dean for Academic Affairs, Friedman School of Nutrition Science and Policy, Tufts University, Boston, USA

Qualification:

PhD in Economic Geography from the University of Birmingham, Birmingham, UK

Focus:

Food security, humanitarian policy and practice, development policy, agriculture and food systems, micronutrient deficiencies and methods of delivery.

Biography:

Dr Webb is former Chief of Nutrition of the World Food Program of the United Nations; a first-responder to the Asian tsunami disaster in Aceh; a member of the International External Evaluation of FAO; member of the UN Millennium Project's Hunger Task Force; former member of the steering committee of the UN Standing Committee on Nutrition.

Dr Webb is involved in research on evidence of impact of integrated agriculture-health-nutrition programs in Nepal and Uganda, policy responses to world food prices; cost and benefits of ready-to-use foods in nutrition programming; evaluation of nutrition programming in Burkina Faso, Malawi, Ethiopia and East Timor; optimal nutrient formulation of food aid commodities; measures of diet diversity in emergencies.

In the past he has worked on such areas as: experiences of famine in Ethiopia and North Korea; tobacco use as displacing food expenditure in Indonesia; optimal design of public works projects in Niger; and tools for assessing household food insecurity in Bangladesh.

Further Information:

http://nutrition.tufts.edu/faculty/webb-patrick

Index

F

C

D

E

F

G

H

I

J

K

L

M

N

O

P

Q

R

S

T

209 **Colophon**

Editorial Board:

Manfred Eggersdorfer
Klaus Kraemer
Marie Ruel
Marc Van Ameringen
Hans Konrad Biesalski
Martin Bloem
Junshi Chen
Asma Lateef
Venkatesh Mannar

**Communication consultancy,
editing and project management:**

Jonathan Steffen Limited
Cambridge, United Kingdom

Design concept, layout typesetting and graphics:

Mark Austin
V-One Design Solutions Limited
Leighton Buzzard, United Kingdom

Proofreading and indexing:

Yvonne Bearne
transparent Language Solutions GmbH
Berlin, Germany